Mental Health Workbook

learn How to Manage Insecurity and Attachment

(Exercises to Transform Negative Thoughts and Improve Well-being)

Mark Postma

I0105998

Published By **Oliver Leish**

Mark Postma

Mental Health Workbook: learn How to Manage Insecurity and Attachment (Exercises to Transform Negative Thoughts and Improve Well-being)

ISBN   978-1-998769-73-5

No part of this guidebook shall be reproduced in any form without permission in writing from the publisher except in the case of brief quotations embodied in critical articles or reviews.

Legal & Disclaimer

Table of contents

Chapter 1: Does Your Personality Affect Your Mental Health?

This chapter has been designed to train you on what persona is and, the way it impacts your mental fitness. So at the quit of this bankruptcy, you are expected with a purpose to discover your character; what is right on your persona; what is not so suitable in your character and how you may improve for your personality with the intention to have a nice mindset to lifestyles and preserve your mental health. You also are predicted to learn the way you may create a tremendous mind-set thru fantastic mind and worldviews.

In various belief systems and non secular circles, if now not all of them, it's miles assumed that what an character in the end seems to be or their persona is decided by means of their day by day confession, utterance, words being utilized by that person in their normal communique, their self declaration and worldview. Therefore in the ones belief structures, humans are constantly cautioned to be cautious and take a look at what they need to mention or would like to mention or how they would act or behave in sure situations. With that during mind, before we cross deeper into understanding what mental fitness is, and the way it could assist one's self attention, we want to understand what persona is.

Therefore, allow me quick take you on a linguistic adventure. I want us to recognize the meaning of the word "persona." To do this, we want to break the phrase down and spot the morphemes that make up the phrase "character." But we have something cogent to do before we do that, and that is knowing the idea referred to as a notion system. Belief machine despite the fact that we aren't going to talk about it significantly in this book, it's far exceedingly affordable for us to recall it as it's far one of indirect foundation on which mental fitness and self focus solidly stand on.

To have a higher understanding of character, we need to first recognize what notion device is. A belief machine is an ideology, indoctrination of precise worldviews or set of concepts which can be most times answerable for the precise interpretation of our regular reality. This, i.E. The belief device may be inside the form of faith, way of life, political leaning, tradition, philosophical thoughts, spirituality, sexuality amongst many other matters. A perception machine is extra dogma than pragma, and it takes real and tangible conviction for it to be changed. Many human beings discover ideas of converting their notion machine repulsive; consequently, they never alternate. Thus, so as to be a better character, you have to recognize your character and inner-self. Personality can higher be visible through what is known as enneagram. Enneagram is a nine-sided figure used to indicate 9 viable persona developments of a subject. So, the total sum of what character becomes is molded and encouraged with the aid of a sequence of different but interconnected elements which comes as a result of your personality kind.

Our expertise on a specific topic and trouble, in which we have been born, the way we had been raised, and even peer stress from friends and pressure from family participants can assist to create and additionally change our character if we make conscious efforts to make our existence higher. It can then be stated that character (i.E. How someone acts or reacts) of an character typically arises from environmental causes and extra awesome in natures; despite the fact that it can be installed one of the nine personalities regarded and those personalities causes are not always formed through organic effects – it comes from nurture and not from nature. The very last convictions and end that come from these systems are a way for us to make meaning of the sector this is unfolding around us and to create our role inside it. So to remember in life, to be privy to personality which we belong and to apprehend the ones human beings that we are accountable to in one manner or the alternative, we want to begin from information our notion gadget, our worldviews and the way we always take the arena will assist us in interrogating anything is thrown at us, and it's going to additionally assist us apprehend our persona. When we try this, we'll be able to have a higher lifestyles, and we can be capable of understand how to take away harmful, poisonous elements and beautify the beneficial factors of our notion device and personality.

Personality has been described as the complexities that come from human conduct and has been visible as all of the capabilities, whether a behavioral, emotional, temperamental, and cognitive state that characterize a completely unique person. This is a noun which incorporates three morphemes: (one free morpheme and sure morphemes) "Person" "al" and, "ity." I will like to speak about 'Person' for now. Many people take individual for the body that's observable, touchable and although shares equal characteristics. Nonetheless, let me burst your bubble, individual isn't like frame, and a person is the overall sum of the persona that an person (body) famous. Taking frame for a person is wrong, individual is distinctively unique from body. For instance, individual(ality) is not physical, but the frame is. The personality, which enneagram is purely approximately, is thought to be complexities that come from human behavior and has been visible as each function, whether or not behavioral, emotional, temperamental, or cognitive country that characterizes a completely unique individual. This consists of imagination, attention, thinking, belief, judgment, language, dress experience, behavior, perspectives, reminiscence worldview, etc. That makeup, define what an person takes himself for and the way the society understand that fellow in question. Personality, for me is some thing which could speedy be defined as the entire sum of individual consciousness and unconsciousness. It is what human beings recognize you to be and the way you deliver your self. To recognize persona, one should apprehend enneagram.

Many dictionaries and books have defined enneagram as a nine-sided discern used to signify 9 viable persona developments of a topic and as the trait of staying aware of (paying close attention to) who you're. This truly approach that personality can also be referred to as the psychological manner of bringing one's attention to every enjoy and things that passed off in the past or is taking place inside the gift second of one's existence. These happenings are what can be said to define that person. So, these items, in the long run, assist an man or woman to turn out to be a unique person/man or woman which can be installed one particular elegance or organization of personalities diagnosed through enneagram of persona.

Personality, on the other hand, is something which you can actually effectively broaden thru the practice of mindful commentary, cautious living, conscious efforts to get better or to keep a few sure behaviors, self-worth or to stay away with a few precise conduct which may restriction one's development and improvement and intellectual increase. Personality also can be advanced through other training and strength of mind. Furthermore, personality within the actual sense, manner keeping a moment-by way of-second awareness of our mind, emotions, physical sensations, and environment, environment, thru a gentle, nurturing lens which facilitates us to become a higher model of who we were on the day past. It follows that when we interact ourselves within the proper act of character development, our mind and feelings emerge as synched with what we're sensing in the present moment rather than rehashing the beyond or imagining the future. So, whilst that is executed continuously, we turn out to be a better individual, and we get to understand different humans in our environment, existence, and surrounding.

From the attitude of neuroscience, a "idea" which on occasion is the inspiration that forms the middle of our personality can be described as a based representation of a factor of view, notion, hypothetical possibility, or meant action which makes up the person which we clearly are. The thought is the type of element that you can write down as a sentence, for instance.

In some discussions and books, it is not but entirely clean, how mind are represented within the mind, however there have to be some form of illustration within the mind that then create a character and make you who you are. In so many books and journals, clues available to this point propose that a few neurons will constitute factors of the idea and others will constitute the relationships a number of the elements.

Working memory probably performs a position in capturing special additives of mind, in order that associative regions of the brain can bind the components collectively. But this is all fairly wild hypothesis based on the clues we do have so far.

It is logically secure to count on that every personality is specific and that each organization in enneagram of persona represents "comparable or assorted thoughts" in one of a kind approaches. One's very own thoughts, worldviews, and character might also represent the same organization of persona in distinct methods. Therefore, as one's thinking evolves, so the arrays of thoughts in us are evolving and which are the elements contributing to our unique character. There are diverse personalities, 9 groups mainly and also you belong to one. Each has its strengths and its weaknesses. You have to pick out and recognize the organization you belong, and while you do, you ought to work on your strength to improve your grit and strengths and ought to usually locate ways to downplay your weak spot in any respect time.

Chapter 2: How To Move Into Your Self Aware And Loving Nature

This bankruptcy is written to reveal you how to circulate into self consciousness state and loving nature s thru know-how of thought and the way advantageous wondering can help you benefit the social standing which you desire. At the stop of this chapter you're expected so one can be capable of apprehend what thought is and the way you can use your idea undoubtedly to achieve great things.

Thought is a totally specific yet interesting phenomenon this is odd to individual. It is believed in one of a kind quarters that thoughts that go through a person thoughts are what outline that individual. We all have thoughts going thought going through our minds at one point on the alternative and we technique thoughts differently which makes us do things in another way at one-of-a-kind factor of our lifestyles. Human being is a considerate being and earlier than we embark on any enterprise we usually try to consider the cease from the start. The end result of our imagination that is our very last notion makes to act, react, or be proactive to an issue handy. This without a doubt shows that we're the feature of our concept and we best exist at a factor in time due to our very last thought. Our thoughts define us.

In our normal existence, it is not unusual to pay attention a person say, "I just had a concept approximately A or C," or "the concept just took place to me." For example, one guy ought to have extraordinary mind about an occasion that occurred over the past World Football Cup Competition. Thoughts may be concept-like in our mind, reminiscence-like, image-like, or tune-like. They are normally don't final lengthy in our thoughts and might exchange earlier than one blinks his eyes. Thoughts are discrete activities and particular to every man or woman, although it is able to be shared, in contrast to non-stop events such as the steady sound of a teach and tick of a clock, notion might be erratic. We, as humans, all enjoy thoughts and we do not have hassle identifying our thoughts and neither can we have trouble speaking about them to our friends, family, coworkers, boss, teachers, therapists and others.

Thought, Self Awareness And Mental Health

From the angle of neuroscience, a "notion" could be defined as a structured illustration of a factor of view, notion, hypothetical possibility, or supposed action. Thought is the form of thing that you could write down as a sentence, for example.

We don't fully apprehend, but, how mind are represented within the brain, however there should be some form of representation. The clues we've thus far advise that some neurons will constitute factors of the thought and others will constitute the relationships most of the elements. The illustration might be relatively dynamic, with millions of neurons firing at exceptional times, and the sample possibly in no way repeats and constantly advances.

Working memory likely performs a position in taking pictures different additives of mind, so that associative areas of the mind can bind the additives together. But this is all fairly wild speculation based at the clues we do have so far inside the area of neuroscience.

Consciousness is the "theatre of perceptual awareness." It's now not clear if consciousness is needed for mind or now not, but it simply allows. Can you've got a thought that you are not privy to? Most humans would say it's now not a thought if so. If you are "lost in notion" and a person asks you what you're thinking and your thoughts "suddenly goes clean", does that mean you weren't wondering anything? If you upward push from your bed in the morning with lucid intuition and perception, does this suggest you had been wondering at the same time as you had been snoozing?

These questions in the end come down to what we suggest with the aid of "concept" in distinct occasions and contexts. We will in the end be able to parent out what goes on in the brain in those extraordinary situations and why; we will then want to determine which kinds of interest we want to name "idea" and which ones not.

Can a single idea be made with the aid of many minds?

It is logical to expect that each mind is precise, and that each mind represents "similar mind" in distinct approaches. One's very own mind can also represent the equal concept in distinctive approaches as one's thinking evolves. What you "apprehend" to be multiplication or a calculus crucial is surely distinct now than whilst you first found out it. The cause is that the building blocks of notion are the representational schemes of the brain - what each neuron represents - and these are converting all of the time because the brain learns.

Chapter 3: Understanding How Others Perceive You

This bankruptcy has been designed to help you apprehend how others understand you. As you examine this bankruptcy, you will be capable of recognize why humans react to you in a specific way and why you constantly get the same reaction from people whenever you are searching for explanation. Also, at the quit of this chapter, you are expected to understand the nexus among character and enneagram and the way you can understand your persona in this kind of way that it will let you end up self aware. You are also anticipated to peer yourself thru other people lens so that you can apprehend how other humans perceive you.

First off, there are four primary personalities which might be well known. These personalities determines how we see your self or see different people and label them. So we on the whole label human beings as phlegmatic, melancholic, choleric, and sanguine. However, consistent with enneagram of character, there are nine precise personalities. According to Ian

Morgan Cron, those are the nine enneagram of persona:

1.   Type One: The Perfectionist.

2.   Type Two: The Helper.

three. Type Three: The Achiever.

4.   Type Four: The Individualist.

five.   Type Five: The Investigator.

6.   Type Six: The Loyalist.

7.   Type Seven: The Enthusiast.

eight. Type Eight: The Challenger.

nine.   Type Nine: The Peacemaker

The Enneagram of persona structure, which I even have also briefly noted in my creation and inside the preceding chapter would possibly appearance sophisticated, however if you open your mind, it's far quite trustworthy and easy to understand. The enneagram of persona is like a tree diagram in which 9 extraordinary specific personalities are drawn. These personalities overlap and once in a while have the attributes of the subsequent one however there are so many dissimilarities between them. These disimilarities are what make the following man or woman see your distinctiveness as being unusual and one of a kind from theirs. So other have a tendency to perceive as you weird due to the fact you are one of a kind from them. You just want to be contented with yourself and not compare your competencies with that of the subsequent one. With comparism comes self doubt, low self-worth, pain, and weakness. Therefore, it's going to help you a top notch deal on a way to understand and totally recognize the character of other humans if you try to draw it yourself. You should additionally create a intellectual photo of the Enneagram of personalities. When you do this, you may be capable of accomplice humans with certain behaviours, and you'll additionally be capable of suit individuals who can have a dating together while not having any thoughts-studying ability or superpower or psyche knowledge. These will absolutely help you in expertise how this world works so you will now not ought to beat your self for being stressed out within the way you're wired.

Your Basic Personality Type

From one particular point of analyzing, the enneagram is visible as a group of nine distinct temperament kind of, with every range at the enneagram denoting one kind. It is not unusual to search out a piece of yourself, altogether 9 of the types, though one in all them should stand out as being nearest to your self. This is your simple character type.

Everyone emerges from adolescence with one from the nine essential personalities dominating their temperament, with inborn temperament and alternative pre-natal factors being the maximum determinants of our kind. This is one component anywhere maximum if no longer all the key authors on persona agreed. Subsequently, this inborn orientation, for the maximum element, determines the approaches which we, people, have a propensity to learn to adapt to our environment and research from our environment.

Furthermore, it additionally appears to persuade, and on occasion stir, subconscious orientations towards our parental figures. However, why that is often so, we do not. Therefore, we will be inclined to nonetheless not hold close what governs our behaviour. In any case, by the point kids are 4 or five years vintage, their focus has evolved sufficiently to possess a separate feel of self. Although their identification is still extraordinarily fluid and oscillating among proper and wrong but they preserve to recognise about the arena around them. At this age, youngsters begin to confirm themselves and word ways of becoming into the social network and the world around them on their personal. This is the procedure that we all went via even as growing up. Hence, we have a tendency to see human beings that are from society or surroundings that is a bit distinctive from us as weird. We locate it tough to just accept them or see them as another awesome character. We choose others and spot them as aberration or deviation from norms because they possess a few traits that are one way or the other one of a kind and new to us.

Thus, the orientation of our temperament displays the totality of all adolescence factors (which include genetics) that stimulated its development. (For a variety of concerning the natural system patterns of every temperament kind, see the related segment inside the kind descriptions in temperament sorts and within the know-how of the enneagram.

We are nearly judgemental with our actions and behaviours so that is why we see others as being not so good as us. So, now which you understand this, it's miles smart for you not to allow the moves of others to decide your happiness or lifestyles. You need to live your existence on your own time. You should develop mentally at your own tempo and also you have to expand a thick skin to grievance. However, you need to note that not all criticism are terrible, the poor ones are terrible and ought to be shut out.

Let us examine some troubles which are germane to character development.

The following factors are very essential to recognise the differences between enneagram organizations

1. People do not surely exchange from one number one character kind to another in a single day.

2. The descriptions of the character types are universal and observe similarly to each genders due to the fact no kind is inherently suitable or bad or female or masculine in nature.

3. Not all matters within the description of your primary type will observe to you on every occasion because you constantly oscillate among the healthy, common, and unhealthy developments that form your persona and types.

4. The character uses distinctive numbers to designate each of the kinds due to the fact numbers are definitely price-neutral.

5. The description of someone or specific persona kinds isn't always full-size at a factor time.

6. No kind is certainly higher or worse than every other kinds, so that you can't say one is higher than the opposite. While all the temperament kinds have distinctive belongings and liabilities, a few types are generally thought of to be a lot of captivating than others in any given tradition or cluster.

In addition to the above, for some specific reasons, you can now not be happy being a selected type due to the negativities attached to it. You may also feel that your type is "confined" in a few approaches. As you research many stuff about all the categories, you will apprehend that just as every has unique capacities in one way or the opposite, every has different limitations. If you study areas, content material, devices, teachings, publications, and discussions on enneagram in a whole lot of prestigious Western society and their faculty, you will see some higher improvement than in other colleges and society. This is due to the characteristics that society decides to reward, not due to any advanced cost of those kinds that we had been discussing up to now. The major idea and purpose is which will improve and become your high-quality self and emerge as a higher version of your self and not to replicate the strengths of every other businesses of character.

Identifying Your Basic Personality Type

Although there are some other software program and social code persona software program to be had in the marketplace via which you may calculate your persona, they are primarily fake. However, there are numerous methods via which you may understand your character without using any software program due to the fact they won't be correct in most instances. This segment is designed, so that you will have a primary know-how of the types in this book while now not having to apply any software or travel to look any psyche, mind reader or study longer descriptions approximately enneagram of personality.

As you watched that regarding your temperament, that which sort of the subsequent 9 roles suits you quality maximum of the time and describe your personality, I am happy to inform you that you will be capable of recognise in which you belong in a short time. Or, to put it succinctly, in case you had been to explain your persona or self in a few sentences, which of the following word clusters could come closest to describing the character you observed you're?

Understanding how human beings view you

These one-phrase descriptors are grouped into 4-phrase units of trends and personalities. Keep in mind and do not forget that those words simply spotlight and don't represent the whole spectrum of every type of enneagram, and the phrases are just to offer a glimpse of who you are.

•   Type One is principled, purposeful, self-managed, and perfectionistic.

•   Type Two is beneficiant, humans-beautiful, demonstrative, and possessive.

•   Type Three is adaptable, excelling, driven, and picture-aware.

•   Type Four is expressive, self-absorbed, dramatic, and temperamental.

- Type Five is perceptive, innovative, secretive, and remoted.

- Type Six is enticing, demanding, accountable, and suspicious.

- Type Seven is spontaneous, versatile, acquisitive, and scattered.

- Type Eight is self-assured, decisive, willful, and confrontational.

- Type Nine is receptive, reassuring, complacent, and resigned.

If you're able to describe your self, you may be capable of know how apprehend view you and thru that you could paintings on your self-worth and personality. You can emerge as higher at what you do.

Chapter 4: How To Downplay Your Weaknesses And Improve Strengths

This chapter will talk approximately how to recognize but in no way settle for your weaknesses. It will, consequently, display you why you must constantly are seeking for improvement on your lifestyles. At the quit of this bankruptcy, you must be able to discover and recognize your weaknesses and strengths. You also are expected with a purpose to paintings on your weaknesses and construct for your power so that you can gain back your self esteem and continuously become self conscious.

It isn't viable which will just turn a weak point right into a electricity in case you are busy downplaying your weaknesses or denying that the weak point exists. Therefore, your first challenge is to renowned that you simply have weaknesses and confirm what they are — weaknesses which are restricting and making you lose the better part of yourself. Weaknesses which are taking a exceptional toll to your self esteem and consuming at your self belief.

For me, my weaknesses are I don't like getting involved in whatever which can make be at direct confrontation with the next man or woman. So occasionally, I observe it from the positive aspect and rather than magnifying my weak spot in that regards, I attempt to see myself as someone who's noticeably dexterous at warding off fighting as a result, I am properly at putting others at function in which they sense at ease any kind they're round me. This has usually positioned me in clever role; but different times caused useless problem. There are oftentimes that I have allow a incorrect trouble and acrimony final too long. This may be because of the truth that I am occasionally reluctant to address and address ugly state of affairs I am no longer pleased with this, but admitting it to myself is useful. It means that I will take this tendency below attention as soon as I am operating on selections regarding what to try and do.

Some years ago, I discovered that four of my friends that I love so much and also accept as true with were actively working to undermine my efforts and government. I felt hurt and betrayed, and while I advised them approximately the issue. I did that no longer inside the open due to the fact I did not need many human beings to be privy to the cracks between us. I discussed the issue with them in digicam a good way to inform me their reasons without any fear. With that, I observed my longstanding-and struggle-avoiding and exercise of retaining the dispute covert.

But I additionally asked for a advice from a actually correct pal that knew both humans and also recognise me too properly sufficient fears unpleasantness abundant, but I do. He cautioned that I should speak with them inside the open. Understand that the dialogue approximately such issue must now not be shied faraway from. He made me understood that discussing the problem within the open will make all of us to talk his thoughts and so we will be capable of get to the foundation of the problem. Knowing that my reluctance to initiate a war of words can also nicely harm me, I gave it a few idea then followed his advice. I delivered the issue to the open once more and this time around all of us discussed openly and got to the foundation of the matter.

So it became proper aspect to do and it turned into a incredible name to take her advice. We took the conflict into the open location helped absolutely everyone to find a closure and I became able to gain a super control over the problems as we all had been able to carry our utmost feelings and idea with a directly face. The count number subsequently died and we persisted our friendship because of the reality that we discussed the entirety in the open and not anything become hidden from every other. This shows that no one is a frame of expertise, you may study from the following individual to be able to end up better at what you do. So do now not ever turn away from in search of the reviews of people who are higher than you in a few approaches.

Embrace Your Mistakes.

Sometimes the only defence towards weak point is to overcompensate with high-quality practise. For example, I even have a feeble experience of course and on occasion generally tend to get lost in my idea, leading to what I will call "intellectual paralysis". I over think issues and then determine now not to take movements over an trouble due to having too numerous options. Sometimes, as a person when you are going someplace, you may discover it difficult to get your approaches. Therefore, I make the most technology to store lots of time, with a GPS for your car, another one on my telephone, and the third one on my pc, anyplace you're you could effortlessly convert the conventional maps online use and find your methods. In some locations in which technology isn't available, you could bring a near paper map additionally so that it will make things smooth for your self.

Similar techniques can be implemented to different things. Are you on the brink of handing out a settlement or taking a proposal with indistinct or unknown terms? Wait a second, analyze scenario and read the whole things earlier than you signal the dotted lines. Ought to pitch a customer for the first time? Learn all you may need regarding the individual you're pitching, then exercise your pitch several times in your colleagues or friends earlier than you ultimately pitch the potential consumer. This way that to get your self esteem and be self conscious on this first century, you have to be prepared and hone your abilities for anticipated possibility. Regardless of wherein you are or what is taking place around you, you have to always have a contingency plan for everything you do so you gained't find your self in a tight nook.

Learn New Skills or Leverage on Other People Skills

Instead of doing one issue you are not clever at, you're happier hiring any person as a way to fill within the talents you lack, both as a contractor or complete time. Besides compensating to your weak spot, this will can help you building up a essential talent you need in locating the workforce you may agree with. When you have recognized their capabilities and strengths, you can leverage them by way of trusting them with belongings you can not do yourself. There is not any reasonable factor in having mistrust on a person whom you're trusting with a mission. So you ought to be prepared to give them loose reign when they're executing the challenge given. It is an indication of indescribable insecurity if you do not agree with a person you're giving a project to complete for you. If you are not certain of someone's competencies or capacities to have the ability to help you reap your preference, you should no longer recruit them in place of giving somebody a venture you do no longer absolutely see them accomplishing.

Always Desire To Learn.

Even even though nobody can ever be sufficient and best every venture, making effort to study, is one way to turn out to be better and enhance your self esteem and become self conscious. When you practice extra on what you do now not recognise, you will get to understand and enhance your self esteem and end up better in life. So it is a great issue to develop a by no means finishing mindset for mastering a this may help you to put your self collectively and get returned at the right tune. A really properly man or woman I as soon as knew headed a digital agency despite the fact that he had no technical talents in that area of interest. Though he agree with his team with the whole lot, he needed and worked difficult to study new talents and advantage enough knowledge concerning what they did to be able to inform after they could have met the requirements and end whatever venture they have before cut-off dates and in the event that they couldn't. So he's able to pick out what became really feasible to do and what was no longer viable for his team to do. As he stated it, he discovered "just enough to attain what is needed at a factor in time."

That is a wonderfully smart approach. There are numerous matters we should all continually be capable of do on our personal. Even if we are not able to do the entirety, we ought to be able to do the basic minimal to a degree. This is because there are a few sense correct feelings that include having the ability to perform a project, regardless of how minute or beside the point such assignment might be. So that is especially true in case you are going to recruit humans as employees and control those who could be running for you. Being able to understand what to do and how to do it, is one way to enhance your self-worth and become self aware in life.

Chapter 5: How To Improve Your Self-Esteem And Confidence

This bankruptcy is designed that will help you understand a way to improve your vanity and confidence. You gets to apprehend tips that could boost your vanity and enhance your self belief if they are well followed.

In a nutshell, shallowness is your opinion of yourself and your capabilities. It may be high, low, or somewhere intermediate at some factors. Whereas absolutely everyone every so often has doubts concerning themselves, low self-esteem will leave you feeling insecure and causeless. You would probable be capable of determine a number of of factors that rectangular measure shifting your opinion of yourself (maybe you're being intimidated, in any other case you could properly be feeling lonely), or it can be a thriller. Either manner, their rectangular degree masses of belongings you may do to boost your self-esteem.

Always be kind to your self so as to do something accurate for your self.

That little internal voice that tells you that you are becoming it proper (or now not) is lots effective than you could possibly consider. Create your own happiness and be type to yourself. If you're slipping, or getting it wrong, make attempt to mission any bad thoughts that is probably crossing your thoughts. The reasonable aspect to do is to speak to your self in the identical way that you would communicate for your buddies or mentees. This can be very difficult on the outset. However, consistent exercise makes you turn out to be accurate and finally turn out to be ideal

Do not examine your self with others.

Comparing your self to others may be a fulfillment, then you may start to sense cheesy. Attempt to without a doubt location your recognition and attention in your desires, objectives and achievements. Instead of comparing your self or measuring yours achievements in opposition to the achievements of other people, try to examine your achievement towards your personal set dreams and no longer against someone else's.

No one wishes that form of strain so do no longer put your self beneath any strain.

Always Be searching for opportunities via exercise your body

Exercise can be an top notch way to extend motivation, practice setting dreams so that you can build your self belief. Breaking a sweat is some other way to help your frame and thoughts with a purpose to unleash endorphins, the texture-true hormones. This hormone can inform on your mind-set, vision in life and can help you gain your confidence returned. So it's far vital which you don't feel dejected continually. You must be accessible running, searching out methods you can improve your very own lot.

Finding inner peace in recent times may be a top notch assignment to you. This is due to the fact the whole thing regarding modern day society sounds like they may be at variance with experiencing peace. It is feasible that you do now not find whatever that makes you experience happy. In such situation, you ought to appearance inwards FOR approaches thru which you may intrinsically inspire your self into getting better. To assist yourself in getting your self-worth, you can do the subsequent:

1.   Focus on matters you could trade

Why fear regarding those things you may't manipulate? It sours your temper and causes you to be less succesful and inactive.

Literally, ask your self, "Is this one issue I will be able to manipulate or manipulate? Can demanding be beneficial in any way? As person, you have got to understand that things are not continually within your manage. There is some thing on the far side that allows you to distract you and vicinity pressure to your life if you do not be cautious.

2. Relate with nature

You must understand people who first exist earlier than us did not sleep in mansion and did no longer possess ranch or devour micro waved pizza. Visit park, walk into jungle, cross trekking and picnic in a few mountains to clean your head. At the end of your revel in and journey, you may feel dramatically totally unique compared to sitting in a completely building twenty-4 hours an afternoon. There's one thing non violent regarding paying attention to birds chirp, looking animals in their herbal habitat time, seeing bushes forming their cover in Amazon forest.

3. Be devoted to your self and do now not pretend.

Nothing is as frightening as residing a life you have been not supposed to live. Faking it till you ultimately make it's miles one manner to get your emotion battered and harm. Living a fake lifestyles regularly put off your existence from you and makes you grow to be demoralized. Live a life that's in tandem together with your values and beliefs. Do now not faux, as living a pretentious can tell on your intellectual health. To have a better self recognition, you have to be in the right body of mind. It isn't a right issue that allows you to allow society or pals to dictate your picks or preference for you. You ought to not to place your life on a career this is simplest interesting to others however now not you. You have to no longer chase a lovely house or costly automobiles because human beings say it is good or lovely however need to constantly are seeking what makes you better and satisfied. Ensure you take rate of your lifestyles via making your non-public selection regarding what is maximum vital to you.

four. Mind what you eat

You might not note how unhealthy you feel due to the fact you are aware of ingesting what isn't precise for your health.

Try eating meals within the manner you recognize you ought no longer to for just a week and jot down the modification and adjustments in how you experience. Analyze meals which help improve your reminiscence, growth your alertness and help you focus and facilitate good feelings. Ensure you handiest devour meals that reason you to sense top and assured about yourself. This is one way through which you may get your mental fitness and be self conscious that allows you to sense assured and satisfied among your colleague. To sense good approximately yourself and get better at what you do, live away from and say no to junk meals and sodas. By cultivating wholesome ingesting dependancy, you may have a better frame construct and super appearance, in the end, this will make a contribution immensely to your standard self belief and self-worth.

five. Exercise daily

Have you ever for once consider how assured you're feeling as you are strolling out of the health club or an interview room after you have got aced it? Exercise feels remarkable and acing an interview or examination feels wonderful, and also you sense exquisite regarding yourself for doing it. Exercise isn't always just for your body, it also facilitates in maintaining your mind healthy. So, as an man or woman running to get your sanity and feel suitable about your self, you have to make effort to exercise every day. By workout, you'll be mentally alerted and equipped for the challenges ahead.

6. Do appropriate deeds and be kind to others

This is a superb way of questioning and helping others in time of want. When you assist humans, you become greater conscious that others are afflicted and want a assisting hand. This lets you cultivate a proper mindset. When you supply happiness to others, you acquire kindness reciprocally. You can even in reality feel a few type of satisfaction and satisfaction once you facilitate someone else's development and happiness. So one certain way to be self aware and benefit your confidence as you live your daily existence is to make sure which you do good unto others and ensure which you have a high-quality attitudes to lifestyles.

The golden rule of life explains that you have to do to different people something you like them to do to you too. This sincerely manner; in case you expect love, provide love, in case you anticipate kindness, be type to different humans as well if you want your to domesticate positive attitude. Always try and facilitate peace and supply admire to everyone around you. This is vital in your mental fitness.

7. Be assertive and opinionated

Be open and assertive with your goals, dreams and needs. People will want to take advantage of you in case you can not be assertive with your desires. One manner to get your mental health in order is to desist from following bandwagon. You need to now not do something because others are doing it. Sometimes what different people are doing isn't the pleasant for you so you can gauge your life based on the expectations of other people. You must set your personal popular and act on it. Give yourself a undertaking to acquire and devote yourself to it. Don't ever permit everyone to reduce to rubble your thoughts or make you sense you aren't appropriate sufficient.

At any factor of your lifestyles have to you let others interfere for your existence affairs, take complete fee of your life. So usually make sure you're up to the venture as you pass in life.

Chapter 6: Meditate Over Your Life

At the end of this bankruptcy, you are expected to learn how to be at peace with yourself thru mediation and conscious living. You should be able to see how you could do an intensive soul looking so one can be assertive and benefit returned your self confidence.

Meditation is so calming and soothing. So meditation is something that could make you spot existence and its attendant troubles correctly. Things are typically now not as they appear. Most instances, what we see is a mirage. So while we eventually get to peer the genuine image, it impacts our mental health and makes us experience down. Meditation will forestall your mind from creating a scenario that appears worse than it definitely is. At a factor while you seem to be doing some thing that is affecting your mental fitness, you need to forestall and appearance inward.

Living one's life with amazing peace is pretty workable if we are ready to put off negativities that typically surround our existence. But to try this we ought to truly be prepared to take a few defining decision and take a few required steps a good way to build the ones things we surely want and turn some mirage to tangible and available truth.

So, to have peace of mind and improve one's relationship calls for meditation and self-love. You want to look at how you relate with others and have to get concerned in meditation and self-evaluation to get your intellectual fitness going. If we are truely honest regarding residing connectedly, wherever we're, we will really sense the real joy of our fantastic emotions. With that, we can never open-heartedly accept our terrible emotions. To hold our sanity and purify our minds off the negativities around us, we are able to choose to apply "micro-meditations" techniques, as suggested by using some professionals to gain the needed changes in our lives.

Micro-meditation can be a tiny amount of focus we are able to easily integrate into our daily lives. It could be a mindfulness-based workout, a breathing method, or a short meditation. After we notice ourselves doing unsightly things and in terrible form, we will mood our reactivity by way of drawing near the issue with open mindedness and with extraordinary warning. Once we are bored, we can re-energize and re-interact our thoughts and awareness at the positive sides of human beings round us and the high quality aspects of our lifestyles too. And once we are satisfied, we will display forth that joy all of the time and end up virtually best in all our dealings.

Mindfulness practice to enhance one's dating with different people is not certainly some other method for purchasing our methods but some thing which could make us enhance and higher in all components of our lives. After we see it totally as a way to understand the specified end result, whether or not or no longer that it reduces stress, create higher awareness, or acts as the best manner of overcoming ennui, we have a tendency to overlook the bigger cause of meditation and mindfulness or conscious living if you want to gain a higher existence for ourselves.

The "micro-meditation" approach asks, "What if you're a obviously compassionate, creative being, and it's simply the strain of always try to perform in some other region this is pretty extraordinary that reasons issues?" we do now not wish to "build" awareness or calm. As individuals, we all want to underplay the underlying instances that are affecting our intellectual health. At that point, we overlook the issue as a coming storm and do no longer upward thrust to the occasion on time. It is crucial that we are calm in each situation but we must additionally see troubles for what they are and be equipped to address them correctly.

With mindfulness and meditation, the intention isn't to squeeze in a really little little bit of heedfulness into your busy existence, as you can a session at the fitness center. It brings existence and calmness into the frenzy of your day-after-day life — the simplest way of expanding the addiction of getting again to our proper selves and making our thoughts pure and loose from hatred is practicing mindfulness and meditation.

Try these micro-meditation sporting activities to consist of heedfulness into your day, each day:

PRACTICE KINDNESS

Best for: alleviating feelings of anger towards others.

"Metta Bhavana" may be a term from the Prakrit language that interprets to be the "cultivation of kindness," within the non-romantic experience. Some edges embrace loads of relaxing over the absence of nightmares, and better attention and readability.

1. Sitting well, take several deep

2. With every exhalation, experience yourself loosening.

three. Ask yourself truely, "Is it viable for me to be glad, should I be, may want to I be cherished?"

four. As you inhale, experience yourself swelling with emotions of calm and kindness.

5. In your thoughts, create an image of somebody with whom you are preventing.

6. Inform that individual, "May you be happy, should you be, ought to you be loved."

7. Create an aura and rays of kindness flowing closer to human beings round you.

PRACTICE BODY SCAN MINDFULNESS

This is some other meditation approach you may use in your self confidence and self attention. When you do a body scan meditation, you stand a great threat of becoming better and creating a effective mindset.

Body scan is useful for freeing emotional emotions of anxiety and frustration.

When you're at loss and don't recognize what to do, this may be accomplished to bring awareness in your body. If you are at work and feeling notably frustrated, you can try this to be inside the nation of recognition and to preserve your intellectual health.

1. Begin together with your toes laid flat on the naked floor

2. Allow them to feel relax and loosen

three. Focus and Specialize your attention to your shins and calves

4. Feel them loosen up and unfasten

5. Specialize your attention to your thighs

6. Feel them relax and loosen

7. Specialize for your buttocks

8. Feel them relax and unfasten

nine. Specialize on your belly

10. Feel it loosen up and unfasten

eleven. Specialize in your chest

12. Feel it loosen up and loosen

thirteen. Specialize on your shoulders

14. Feel them loosen up and loosen

15. Concentrate on your palms and palms

sixteen. Feel them relax and unfasten

17. Specialize to your neck

18. Feel it relax and unfasten

19. Finally, cognizance your interest to your face: your lips, nose, eyelids, and brow.

20. Feel all relax and loosen

FOCUS ON AWARE COMMUNICATION

This is the nice method for handling life and for creating conversations with ourselves and others.

In her book which become titled "Real Happiness at Work" and which changed into designed for readers to discover their motive in existence, Sharon Salzberg indicates doing those three matters each time we tend to get stuck in robust conversation that may need to tell on our feelings:

1. Become wakeful to our bodies: this lets in us to gauge our body-language and also the things we would do unknowingly. It moreover

approach we can be capable of gauge the feelings we're experiencing.

2. Use the "I" language: when we use that we need to take advantage of the expression, "I feel….", we tend to create problem for our companions while we argue with them. We feel our power dissipating and make the scenario becomes an atmosphere in which warfare prospers.

3. Be honestly unsleeping to what the following person is announcing: after we're relaxed, this turns into less complicated. Once listening with complete awareness, the subtext of what we are hearing can usually turn out to be obvious. This means that to recognize what takes place around us, we need to be calm and attentive.

PRACTICE BELLY RESPIRATION

Best for: Handling disturbing feelings.

Belly respiratory is exquisite for handling bad emotions. When you feel disappointed, area one hand on your chest, and additionally the closing hand in your stomach. You are making an try to breathe, unforced, in a really ideal manner. That manner you are restricting the motion of the hand for your chest, so it is sincerely your stomach it's doing the rising or puffing and falling.

According to Loch Kelly, you can enhance your shallowness in case you get your self concerned in meditation. Kelly maintained that to emerge as self aware, one may also take a look at meditation via the following:

1. allow your cognizance to manoeuvre from reading phrases to listening to the sounds around you.

2. make effort to shift from hearing sounds to focusing your interest at the matters round you, staring at object without any tangible form which are all situated all round you.

3. rest and let your mind be at peace into this silent alert cognizance.

Gaining Mental Health By Practicing Eyes Awareness

1. With a tender gaze, merely see what are clearly in reality there ahead of you.

2. Notice the matters which can be unfolding via your eyes and to your presence.

three. Currently close your eyes and spot an equal cognizance that was searching remains here.

4. Visualize correct things and be satisfied

As I stated within the previous bankruptcy, finding peace in this present day world, wherein corruption, lies, wars, preventing, failures, and different poor matters are happening day by day, is like finding a needle in a haystack. But there are many reasonable approaches to keep inner peace.

A best way of acquiring expertise and self-upkeep is how our brains in cooperation with our minds, are mostly stressed out to grasp to the past and forgotten events of our lives. They every now and then carry our past (whether high-quality or terrible) to the fore. When that is executed, the unsightly past that we had starts offevolved to haunt us and prevent us from reaching our goals. It also prevents us from accomplishing our potentials with the aid of exposing us to wrong aspects of our lives. We consciously or subconsciously normally hold connected to profound stories – visceral feelings that linger despite the fact that they will not be in our pursuits.

Remembering those past studies may also be beneficial to you at some other time. However, experiencing them at yet again through our creativeness is surely nurturing a festering and but to be healed accidents and heartbreak that finally provides no value to our present existence and situations.

What time did you feel alive and while final did you experience happy and joyous? At what time did you understand yourself to be smiling and satisfied for no precise reasons? Do you even hold in mind the last time your coronary heart turned into complete of completely happy?

You see, when you are clinging to the toxic past, I am telling you, you're doing nothing however stripping your self of happiness and the possibility to enjoy a brand new feeling and proper things that can make you increase in existence.

Clinging tightly for your pasts can be said to be a really perfect end result of a self-doubt, limiting beliefs, warped wondering that always confuse you that the poor event of your past or something that changed into finished to you through someone else, or what you furthermore may did to your self can be the determining elements of how your lifestyles as a completely unique man or woman will cross or give up. That is a lie, your past do not actually define you. Even though your beyond can be said to be a part of your general identification, yet it does not determine what you become in lifestyles. And the issue and bad times that you are currently experiencing and suffering with cannot cross till you to permit cross of that beyond and consciously decide to be a better person. So you've got your destiny to your hand and you may make it what you need it to be.

Holding on to the harm and ache of the past which you went through isn't always the quality aspect to do. Therefore, you must placed on a fantastic appearance and right power so you can obtain your aim and feature the persona that you so choice. When you often try this i.E. Keeping to the hurtful past, you're doing nothing but shooing and chasing away the fine things that you may have. You are also blocking off channel via which effective feelings and balanced worldviews can come in and reshape your existence.

This hurtful beyond may be the heartbreak you suffered within the past, the lack of a person so pricey to you, betrayal from close allies, transgression out of your workers or the issue of assault on your u . S . And bad results that that attack always brings on your coronary heart on every occasion you consider it. It would possibly also be betrayal and love misplaced between fans, allow us to say among you and your female friend or boyfriend.

I need you to recognize that not until you decide to return head to head with what came about and face the scenario head-on, you'll not be capable of gain your heart goals or have a higher persona or relationship with other humans. You have to cleanse your thoughts of the harm and must make your heart come to be pure and purify it from all hatred, harm which might be drawing you lower back on your adventure to self-discovery and higher living. You should mend your hurtful beyond and deal with the wounds, injuries and awful matters so you may be able to deliver light into your once gloomy global as you pass on in existence and development to the subsequent stage of your life. All those matters which can be still persevering with to hang-out you have to be decisively handled.

You ought to reconcile your beyond and gift and need to reconcile your destiny with your past sooner or later in life. When you do this you may be able to put your lifestyles at the right song. It begins with making excellent selections. Exert the mental consciousness and consciously choose some thing better and ought to duly keep on the emotions that reason you to be satisfied in any respect time if you actually need to be the happiest individual you preference to be.

You are hoarding low electricity within you and need to get rid of them. When you stretch a volute spring, it hoards electricity interior. And as you try and arch it and release it at its seams, the power inside is also duly launched and driven into the a ways distance where it can not be recovered. Like that, this is how you are. You have to be clinical and tremendously intentional with the whole thing you do and have to be ready to live according to your very own time period. Your life must be lived inside the way you want to stay it now not in the manner that others predicted you to stay.

By preserving onto the terrible feelings and hurtful beyond that were as a result of the undesirable events that took place for your beyond, you maintain the terrible power within yourself. But when you unharness the spring and relinquishing the negative vibes, you provoke an emotional detoxification procedure inside you. You start making the needed peace with your beyond, and as you are doing that, you are also becoming a better and progressed personality.

When you reconcile along with your past by using eliminating terrible matters in your past, you produce an entirely new feeling of general and authentic freedom. This freedom is a spoil from poor vibration and emotions, freedom to forgive your self of your wrongdoings, and many different things which you are not so happy with. Thereby, when you try this, you get the freedom to recalibrate yourself, reenergize and actualize your visions, ambitions and the most sizeable potentials that you never suppose may be unleashed.

Steps on the manner to reconcile your beyond with destiny

Step 1: Desist from recollecting poor pasts, no matter how painful they are.

I will tell you the naked truth: Letting pass isn't always an clean thing to do. It requires sacrifice and firm decisions. You may also anticipate it's far simply a count number of placing the past wherever it belongs, ruminating over it, and as a way to do it in the long run, it is never so. It requires predominant work and conscious efforts.

Let me let you know, letting go of the beyond isn't easy a all the ones. It is an exhausting task. Those 5 minutes motion pictures and podcast which you listen to or typically watch on YouTube, Facebook, TV and other media aren't surely the case. The video are made with soundtracks and visuals which can be designed to show you twenty, ten 5 etc. Smooth ways to cope with your beyond. While the ones formulae may want to ease matters by using appealing in your senses and emotions, there are so many methods which can be a ways greater higher. Also there are a lot of statistics that this video are hoarding from you which might be simply tough to do and are components of the processes that they are showing. What i imply is that the films on social media on the way to address your beyond best show you the tremendous factors of life but fail to reveal you the entire picture of what is required to reap your goals and intentions. I, myself determined the ones hints the difficult way even though and need to assist you to know. The extra I tried to shove the past far from my recognition, the more constantly it became and the extra stubbornly it refused to move.

So, what I sooner or later got here to apprehend as I attempted tough to let pass of my beyond is that placing my beyond trauma and hurts away is the worst thing I could do.

Instead, I determined to allow myself move returned to all the ones painful reminiscences and take a look at them and notice why they befell to me. What I did become that I enabled myself to grieve – grieve my unmet goals, and each of these shivery and nervous moments I was compelled to try this, which I could not simply manage as a touch baby simply growing up.

That become so hard to behave out for me. Because for me, going via hurtful past with the aid of revisiting the hurtful and painful moments, pasts or intervals of your life you begin finding resolution and option to the hurts. You will see a totally first-rate restoration transformation happening to you right away. This is precisely what remedy for mental fitness and intellectual balance is genuinely all approximately despite the fact that we are not going deeper into that in this e book.

Jean Jenson, the famend creator of Reclaiming Your Life, installed that we ought to decide to revisit our past even though that beyond brings ache, harm and bad emotions with it. When we do this, we can be capable of make the wanted peace with the past, we can be able to grow and improve our lives then we will be able to assist others who're presently dealing with what we handed through. So for your mental health, it's miles essential that you look backward to recognize what mistakes you made inside the beyond. It is likewise crucial to apprehend what's sincerely dragging you back and what you need to do to avoid the pitfalls you recognized out of your beyond. When you recognize everything about yourself, you could be intentional about your choices and alternatives in destiny.

As she wrote in some other e-book of her – "When revisiting youth things, you could enjoy a incredible deal of agony. Allowing that to occur— weeping once your tears waft is everyday and welcomed, crying out loud and displaying the feeling isn't always something terrible, "seeing" your on the spot or extended circle of relatives individuals, being "back there wherein you have been" as you visualize it, being "inside the frame" of the kid you were— makes it a completely easy task for the electricity of the helpless toddler's unfelt and untapped pain to start flowing via your thoughts, undefended undiluted, unchecked and untouched. When this happens, you end up self aware, healing start occurring for your lifestyles and your mental fitness now become some thing wonderful and super for the type of life you need to live.

You can suppose that such issue will retain for ever. No, it will cease. What you skilled "back there" now begin to be lucid to you. You come to be aware, and it all appears greater lucid and clear to you right away. When this sort of scenario arises, then you get realize those that you ought to installed area in an effort to avoid the pitfall and sooner or later grow to be higher at something you do.

For me, I also used to pen down the situations and hurtful conditions that I need to keep away from in life and the way I am going to react when confronted with those conditions. I also write those matters I want and the way I am organized to reap them and the way I am going to obtain them with little or no help from different human beings.

After writing down all of the studies that I need somewhere in a white easy paper, I would possibly have clearly forgotten the matters that I wrote down at the paper even though the ones matters are looking at me. This is due to the fact, I need to dedicate them to coronary heart and make certain that they go away the face of the papers and get to my thoughts, my entire being and that those words written down come to be a part of my fact The truth that turned into written are now and again simply there, completely exposed to me, but not anything would be accomplished about them due to the fact I might have failed sooner or later to take the necessary step that is reconciling my beyond with the existing.

Chapter 7: How Can You Find Inner Peace?

Finding inner peace is what you could do, and this bankruptcy has been designed to explain how you can do that in a quick time. However, earlier than you discover inner peace you ought to make peace with your self, your lifestyles, your destiny and whom you have been in the past due to the fact this is where it has to begin from. To achieve inner peace and enhance your mental health, you should take the following steps:

Step 1: Highlight the negativities around you.

When you have got time off, without telling each person, just make attempt to visit a totally quiet location. When you're in such area listing, in super info, all of the objects that had hurt you inside the past and are still hurting and haunting you. Do that for all of the beyond activities that you may don't forget up until the present day day of your existence. Do now not force some thing if it does no longer manifest to you evidently. You ought to do that if this is the most effective alternative that you have left.

Putting those precise occasions on paper might be a way which may take a second to endure. You might turn out to be crying during the day for no logical reason. You might also grow to be depressed. You may not be as productive as you need to be at your process.

Know that this is all proper and it will definitely help you improve your mental health. Do not try to rush and never try to conceal your feelings. Neither have to you do anything to result in it or recover from it. Let yourself linger over the painful past. You can twiddling your thumbs, writhe your frame, exhale, sigh or simply allow the emotion out as you do. Do no longer hide your feelings, allow them to come out evidently. As you start to write down the whole lot about your past with overall honesty, you need to have the sensation to be inclined over again to the matters that can reason you ache. As you do that, the comfort and happiness that you choice will come to you evidently within a short time.

Step 2: Decide to embrace your beyond no matter how hurtful it's far.

Just as I stated inside the previous chapter, you must allow cross of hurtful feeling. By identifying to refuse to include your past, you aren't doing something however arguing with the stark truth. When you have critiques as "I desire I had been now not born to this own family but do some other one" or "I desire my mother and father had greater useful sources to make my lifestyles higher" you are ruining the complete method because you are not virtually doing some thing which could haste your healing procedure and facilitate your development. It has in reality taken me extra years and time to nurture the idea of embracing things the manner they are.

My childhood period and developing up turned into any such disturbing enjoy that I do no longer usually like to do not forget. First of all, I lost something so close and dear to me when I turned into so little and could not were extra superior in age. I became younger and what I misplaced turned into so painful because it become so precious to me for my part irrespective of what other humans assume. I additionally continuously consider many days that my mom laboured so hard to make me glad or to peer me through. So anytime I keep in mind those things, I always turn out to be so faint-hearted, however I could not allow my hurtful past outline me. Therefore, I constantly take my thoughts off the ones bad matters to alter myself to the modern-day state of factors.

When that element that I simply informed you about was misplaced, my entire international came crumbled quickly. Emotionally, for decades I struggled to locate my toes, and usually have reasons to grieve and mourn the loss of that prized asset of mine. That aspect almost defined my complete world, however I did now not permit it to outline me.

But I need you to apprehend that after I finally became myself. I began to forestall bringing that hurtful beyond to my present fact for nothing but as an alternative use the beyond to guide me in making selections for my gift instances and futures. Furthermore, as I persevered to ponder on the events and what I even have handed via in my existence, I commenced to look those hurtful activities for what they in reality were even if they had been no longer something I simply preferred. The fact become that, as I began doing that, I in the end became relieved and freed from my pressure. So, as you know, become aware of and understand your persona, you have to reconcile your beyond with the existing if you actually need to turn out to be better in existence.

For years, it became in my dependancy to be resisting to those matters that had already came about to me and cannot be modified or modified. This restricted my development and improvement, despite the fact that I later have become conscious and altered. Now, I don't handiest block out terrible matters in my lifestyles, I use them to my personal benefit.

I am not advocating romanticizing the struggling of your upbringing. I know bringing that to fore can reason great mental effect and ache.

Just like I noted in the preceding chapter, no matter what the keenness or power and mind you make a decision to region into it, the past will not be changed and could handiest continue to be the same. Making peace with your self and beyond is some thing this is critical and should be finished. You ought to take the beyond for what it became and need to consciously determine to become higher as you flow on.

Accepting your beyond in place of repressing your beyond will create a excellent remedy on the way to prevent your future from turning into an limitless struggle. So, the best possibility of the usage of your past to come to be self aware is to merely settle for what it changed into, no matter how awful it in reality was.

Step 3: Find the best in each scenario

There is a hidden treasure altogether in our experiences. This may be difficult to check to begin with, but when you situation your mind to emerge as at peace with past pain, you're allowing your self to get hold of the useful and profitable possibilities in preference to just merely sulking inside the negativity.

Hardship can serve you in beneficial ways, as properly. An terrific initiative for conditioning your thoughts to usually be at the look is by means of writing down the ones desirable things you want in existence. I inspire you to start off listing all of the beautiful things that came out of your ache and begin growing peace together with your beyond.

Step 4: Stop Thinking of What Could Have Been

To make peace along side your beyond, you are probably trying to exchange what has already befell. Well, this approach does now not actually paintings.

Our most important explanation for our suffering takes place as a result of the fact that we will be predisposed to attach restricting beliefs to our past. Most of the proscribing beliefs are available in forms of need to have and shouldn't have. Such as-

"My boss and co-workers must have given me due respect."

"My ex-husband or boyfriend must no longer have betrayed or stabbed me inside the back."

"My ex-wife or lady friend should no longer have betrayed or stabbed me in the back."

Whatever took place within the past already happened? Therefore, brooding over feasible situations that could have played out "should have/ought not" to were isn't going to give you the wished alleviation you're looking for.

When you assert things like "my father or my mother or my boss, or my colleague etc, must have respected me," this form of thinking completely creates suffering and it makes you now not see the hassle out of your perspective but as different human beings's fault. You ought to look inward and understand that It ought to have passed off exactly the manner it virtually occurred. You understand why? Because that become exactly the way it passed off.

A superb and possible method of reconciling your past with your present situations and situations might simply be like this, "My father behaved in a way he did due to the truth that he became sporting his very own ache, negativity, insecurities and detrimental

74

acquisition which were killing him however he could not share with each person. It could be beautiful, implausible and nearly out of location or even weird if, notwithstanding all of his problems and what he became dealing with, he still selected to deal with me with respect, regards and dignity".

I are aware of it by no means helped me, no matter the number of instances I told myself, "My pal have to understand and act kind in the direction of me." Well, she ought to be the perfect person she became at the time as a result of that's the manner she become. In my lifestyles, I observed that what caused me the suffering turned into my idea of how I used to trust she must or have to now not have behaved in a specific way.

Step five: Don't trouble approximately who angry you

Many humans are stuck inside the past notion that recognition and acknowledgment of the hurt and ache you will ease your pain and you may eventually turn out to be detoxified of the hurt and hatred. You count on that the wrongdoer will sooner or later acknowledge their mistake and express regret. This may not show up. So you want to brace your self up and act out the life you choice.

Why might you sit yearning for an apology from any person who changed into the one that even brought about you the ache at the beginning vicinity? You do no longer assume that character who poisoned your pricey pizza to return lower back and notice you lying useless within the health center. I bet you don't need such character around you. Do you want that? I am very certain you do now not need that to occur. So you do now not want to count on apology from someone who hurt you. If they do apologize in reality, excellent, and in the event that they fail to achieve this, there is no purpose for alarm.

You may also desire to pay attention to these words from your real determine- "I grasp I used to incorrect. I made severa errors and wrong selections. I can now feel your ache and grasp you are sincerely hurt by using me. I'm therefore sorry". Nonetheless, as much as you need these words to be said to you, this word might not be really said to you. This is because lifestyles isn't like that. Something we in no way trade and it is left to you to find a closure.

The man or woman who hurt you is perhaps now not enlightened sufficient to supply you with the wished closure which you are seeking for. So, ask your self actual, "Why am I urgently looking for this from that fellow?"

Another man or woman's validation and acknowledgment will now not help your emotion and healing method so that you ought to no longer are looking for social approval from humans. Establishing peace and reconciling your beyond along with your gift and destiny is definitely up to you. The validation of someone else and social approval will now not lead you to wherein you want to get to. You should recognize your personality kind and use it for your benefits.

The proscribing perception of "I want you to understand the hurt you caused me" truely continues you within the radius of pain and self-harassment.

As a remember of fact, you do now not need them to acknowledge your ache. You might be able to patch up collectively with your past even while you do not have their acknowledgment and forgiveness.

Step 6: Forgive and not to mention

You can't start to form peace collectively with your beyond till you forgive. Forgiving is all regarding you and has not anything to try to with the person who has dedicated a transgression against you.

Ask your self even as now not judgment – "how am I proscribing myself by holding onto all of this negativity closer to this character or enjoy?"

Yes, I get it. You are feeling such loads of hatred and gall closer to that person or individuals who have hurt you. Let me tell you, that is not fine in your mental health as you do not want to pay evil with evil. I was once there too. However, keep in mind which you truely forgive for you, now not for her, him or them.

Forgiveness is one in all all the hardest matters to attempt to do. However, certainly forgiving is absolutely an advantage. It isn't always vital to shape peace collectively together with your beyond. It is certain that this stuff are going to be helpful in your boom. However, you may be capable of even patch up together together with your beyond.

Chapter 8: How To Face Your Past And Step Toward Healing

This bankruptcy is designed to teach you how to move ahead in lifestyles. At the cease of this chapter you're predicted to be able to listing how you can eliminate hurts and majestically step into your restoration.

You can not step toward your recovery with the aid of preserving on to the hurtful emotions and grudges of the beyond. So, what do you need to do? This chapter will give an explanation for and give you recommendations on a way to face your past and step in the direction of recovery right away. It will even give an explanation for what it intended to be healed and to get over your beyond. It is apparent that going through the past is not very easy to do, but one has to do it to analyze and grow.

When making a decision to maintain on to past grudges, you surrender yourself to different human beings's whims and caprices. You also are subjecting your self to pain, bitterness, hatred, and dangerous emotions, which can restrict your achievement. This could even smash your future and make you lose cognizance of your imaginative and prescient and future. In addition to that, you may start to deprive yourself essential happiness and peace of thoughts that you rightly deserve.

Stay conscious and be aware as soon as terrible mind and feelings arise. Allow them to return and move as they please, and don't suppress them. Staying conscious of every passing notion could be very important.

Assume you are in your can riding in the useless of night time, and vivid headlights are shining at you at every direction. Your eyes are pressured on any or all of these lighting, and it takes a few attempt to now not confirm them and wonderful and powerful those lights are. However, to continue forward, you want to make certain you attention to your methods and where you're using. You need to endure in thoughts that the distractions which you are seeing will not get you in your destination, but while you are targeted and capable of discover or pressure your manner via, you may be capable of get to where you're going to with out something stop you.

Do no longer allow your self to turn out to be absorbed by means of all the lights that shine on you. Instead, be aware them, and gently look into your desired awareness purposefully. Within the case of a motive force, this means staying on your lane – keeping heading within the proper route. And once you're heading in the proper course, you may in reality be capable of produce what you desire out of every notion that passes through your thoughts in short succession.

You can decide to channel your teach of mind into creating peace together with your beyond by using swing the stress on mind that serve your recuperation system and make you a better man or woman. You can take the following steps to step into your restoration:

Create a desire that permit you to definitely deal with the past

Making peace together with your past wishes you to consciously decide you are capable of do, consequently. It is set realizing which you are bored with reliving that beyond each single day. Decide at once which you aren't attempting to preserve the past.

You would possibly want therapy. And it conjointly might also take time to seek out the proper healer that in reality gets you.

But when you've created up your mind, you're inclined to prevent protecting directly to the beyond, then this could be an awesome starting. This is essential for your intellectual health.

Harness your subconscious to face your beyond so that you may be healed.

Sometimes, as we generally tend to maintain trying what we preference and sit up for, we have a tendency to nevertheless want to assist our thoughts to give you new thoughts and to form peace with the beyond. There aren't any different methods we can use to get our existence returned on track than subliminally creating fantastic situations in our mind. Our subconscious mind may be tuned to assist advocate ways via which can create best manner out of the maze and quagmire that we discovered ourselves. Doing that, we will subliminally dig deep to the foundations and reasons at the back of each downsides of our harm and break ourselves unfastened.

In some days, you are possibly feeling this disappointment and negativity without even knowing what precipitated it. It may be a odor of 1 issue, a TV advert, or radio jingle, any person inside the road that resembles the person who hurt you. Possessing a tremendous level of reasoning skills can virtually move a long manner in developing your character. Not all and sundry is so lucky enough to be born with a silver spoon so many needs personal sacrifice and area to chart their very own path and make their life better. However, the coolest component about all this is the fact that being a higher person is something manageable when you have your mind-set on it. If you persist and apply the right regulations that worked for other achievers and a success human beings you'll clearly be able to keep the stability and come to be higher. What you want is to imbibe the private abilities and observe the success recipe in each day of your lifestyles. When you wake inside the morning, you must have your responsibilities properly set out and need to constantly have quick- and long-time period desires which you really want to obtain. Once you have finished the quick time dreams, you should in no way lose awareness at the lengthy-term desires as so as to be the main element that may make you higher to your lifestyles.

You should always are looking for know-how and understanding as the ones matters will immensely contribute for your goals and lifestyle. Your total education, way of life, worldviews, and professional life-style have something to do with your dreams. The abilties you have acquired within the beyond are also germane to having the existence you need. Therefore, it is not simplest beneficial however important which you paintings so hard to benefit information and sellable talents. You have to appearance the way that the sector is drifting and try and locate stability or learn competencies that can make you relevant within the world.

Having a few particular method and viable techniques up your sleeve and toward the development of your sellable capabilities and useful information will pass a protracted manner in getting your coronary heart dreams. For you to reap the set goals, you must do not forget and make use of these following wide but associated factors of your cognitive notion technique and worldviews. These are a number of it:

(1) Renewing your notion sample for an entire new one

(2) Jolting your critical and analytical thought pattern so you can emerge as better.

(three) Identifying the thought that isn't always potential and appears highly illogical

Since when you had been younger, exclusive happenings and social expectation were wiring and programming you to assume and behave in some real ways. While your primordial intuition will constantly play leading function to your mind-set and reactions to how a particular scenario is handled, you can then redefine and software your thoughts to be careful of the exchange and the way your thoughts act and system some problems at a factor in time. What is discussed below will come up with the wished idea approximately what I am talking approximately.

Ruminate on Why and the Reasons Behind Every Situation

Know and separate the motive and motivation that govern your ordinary moves and worldview from those spontaneous motivations. Furthermore, you ought to always ensure you do no longer lose attention of your lengthy-time period goals and purposes. After that, you ought to always try to work towards your goals via continuously ruminating on what must be completed and the path you have to take if you are to fulfil your dreams and gain your intentions with out a restrictions.

Always Be Cognizance of the Consequences of Each of Your Actions

You should continually try to envision the possible consequences (both effective and negative) of each choice of yours. You have to evaluate the decisions and alternatives you are making or the ones ones that you are choosing no longer to make. You need to use your reasoning ability to create one of a kind eventualities of the feasible outcomes, both positive or negative consequences. This, in a way, will no longer handiest help you to apprehend the worst-case and first-class-case scenarios however can even make you have the ability know the possibly responses and opportunities available to you in every state of affairs.

Identifying the thought that is not attainable and appears fairly illogical

The predominant goal in the back of this is to widen your mind and wondering styles. Like your actual physical frame, your thoughts calls for exertion and exercising as properly to characteristic optimally and assist you obtain your desires and visions. For that cause, you could comply with the pointers which can be given under.

You Must try to Learn Something New Every day

To preserve your thoughts and make it pristine or properly cultivated, your thoughts wishes to be fed with some thing new that it has by no means been fed in the beyond. Whatever you need to feed your thoughts must be some thing useful and educative as this is the simplest manner through which you may broaden and enhance. Keeping your mind charged with riddles and new ideas is one of the first-rate methods via which you could enhance your cognitive capabilities and powers. Through that, your mind turns into sharp, and you'll be in a position to persuade how you think and how people around you act or react to problems. To try this correctly, you need to make certain what you are deciding on to invest your time and mind on is something that comes from new and unusual domain due to the fact this is the manner to preserve your thoughts curious and continue to be sharp.

Create a Choice to Totally Deal With the Past

Making peace along side your past wishes you to consciously determine you're capable of do, therefore. It is about realizing which you are tired of reliving that past every single day. Decide immediately which you are not allowing the past to outline your future.

You may need remedy. And it'd occur which you do no longer discover the right man or woman to help together with your therapy consultation. I need you to apprehend that such situation have to no longer deter you from studying precise books and surrounding your self with humans with positive minds. This will assist and make you gain your lifelong dreams. So studying true books and being round those who can lift your spirit up may be an excellent starting.

Getting Better

In today's age of virtual media and handheld devices, physical workout is generally getting out of hand, as many people use for machines for even simple obligations that could help them get physically healthy and great. It is tested that a healthy frame can house accomplice expeditiously working brain. Besides, schooling and exercising cast off strain and fear out of your existence. It additionally decreases your anxiousness and all your issues. Try to consist of physical pastime to your day by day habitual and make sure it's far covered in you should gain each day purpose if you really want to enhance your cognitive degree and get the nice from your personality and make use of your persona in a resounding way

You Must Keep a Detailed and Balanced Diary

Writing specified each day sports into a dairy will not simplest help your remembrance and reference competencies however will as well, facilitate a upward push on your reasoning skills and habits. First of all, it allows you to go again on your day and spot how you may have performed it higher or in any other case. It also offers the possibility of self-exam and reflection at the selections made or forgone, your movements or inactions. It also shows you your final selections at certain factor of your life.

This, in a way, improves your concept method and keeps track of the development, self discovery that you need to have duly created and the picks you made at that point in time of your development and self-discovery.

You Must Read Good Books

As the age-long aphorism goes, "Books are the ingredients for your thoughts." Books normally, both non fiction and nonfiction prepare you for the inevitable surprises that we may want to encounter in real lifestyles. Moreover, you come to be acquainted with the meant "grey areas" that we have a propensity to stumble upon in our lifestyles. To quote, "you live simply as soon as; however, books reason you to stay thousand lifetimes."

Create a Mental Fitness Routine

There are without a doubt two sizeable strategies wherein to assemble a intellectual health habitual:

Balancing tasks/sports to ensure all intellectual "muscle groups and neurons" are truly being labored intensely. Setting aside time to hit the mental health club with activities best for the intention of constructing wit, robust intelligence and reasoning competencies is good to your intellectual health and self attention.

Chapter 9: Embrace Who You Truly Are

Fear of rejection and failure are sizeable troubles for special human beings in life and it was once for me too until recent time. I was the type that would be so concerned approximately how other humans felt approximately me or how they understand me. This, more often than now not frequently make nervous and traumatic in my interactions with the people mainly the ones I am assembly for the primary time. I continually strive so difficult to constantly say, do and act within the "right" manner and attend to problem so that they would love me being an American or at least count on I am an ideal character and have a groovy character.

What I did not recognize in those years was that there have been some methods I was rejecting myself, which led me to feel like I changed into now not true. I become searching out outer validation and people's validation. My worry of others' rejection became a projection of the numerous ways wherein I was rejecting myself unknowingly.

That turned into what befell many years in the past from now. Fortunately, when I placed a forestall to rejecting myself and started out embracing who I become, my fear of others' rejection went away effects.

In working with numerous heaps of human beings of various sun shades, shade and creeds with different aims and personalities for many years, and in recuperation my very own persona deficiencies and in handling my personal worry of rejections.

1. Judging Yourself Harshly

Do you sense down and unhappy or unworthy whilst other humans decide you, specially when they misjudge you or your intentions? If yes, the same thing occurs whilst you decide yourself however simply that it happens at the unconscious stage, that you cannot physically see however mentally perceive. Self-judgment could be a common and powerful style of self-rejection.

Are you tuned in to the way you experience as soon as you make a decision to do some thing for your self without traumatic about the consequences? Or have you ever numbed out your feelings, that's every other not unusual shape of self-rejection? Are you conscious that once you choose your self, you feasible experience tense, depressed, guilty, ashamed and/or angry? Have you ever linked those emotions directly to your self-judgment and condemnation?

If you were to decide one little child by means of saying words which includes, "You are so pathetic," "You are the maximum stupid," "You are so unpleasant and now not worth of every person's care or interest," "There is some thing mainly incorrect with you," "You are not and could in no way be true enough for anything," By announcing that you are passing a totally incorrect judgement. The same component happens while you choose yourself. If you imagine which you without a doubt are levelling these judgments toward a touch child among you, then you'll truly be capable of start to draw close why judging your self may be a selected fashion of self-rejections and self-condemnation.

2. Ignoring Your Feelings

Many parents grew up studying to ignore our painful emotions because of that we will be predisposed to manage them negatively. One positive manner for lots of us to learn how to not sense our pain and harm is by way of disposing of our mind from our bodily frame. At that level, we only want to put our minds on something high-quality and attention on it. This isn't always denial however high quality thinking that may help us plenty. You place your mind wherein your frame is not due to the fact your emotions and emotion are extraordinary from logics and while each thoughts and frame that is wherein the feelings are within the identical vicinity you may find it difficult to assume definitely or constructively. You must positioned your awareness for your mind in place of your frame or the hurtful beyond. But even as actual kids can feel rejected in case you ignore their emotions, the kid among feels rejected when you forget about your emotions. The internal kid is your feeling self, therefore once you keep for your mind and disconnect from your feelings, you are rejecting a vitally essential facet of your self that's harmful.

You can virtually forestall your self from rejecting your self in any respect time. You can learn to take price of your existence and be chargeable for your personal emotions and actions. You can begin to speedy control your ache and hurtful emotions. That is exactly what I needed to learn how to do in a few ways. I found out it, and it's miles assisting me grow and increase to what I intend to be. I consider all people can expand and rise if they so decided to achieve this. I love developing and stepping beyond boundary set with the aid of the society, so that is what I essentially assist my buddies, people and absolutely everyone round me do, and that is what hundreds have learned to do through training self-love and via seeing larger version of themselves. When you discover ways to like yourself instead of rejecting your self, then you'll be able to certainly proportion love with others, rather than constantly trying to get love and keep away from the pain of rejection.

Furthermore, self-love is something that everybody desires but finds it difficult to define or hold close. Therefore, Self-love although is a popular term today it usually receives twisted in everyday verbal exchange. People generally say: "You need to like your self a lot" "Why don't you like your self?" "If you adore your self, see your self as a favourite, and additionally see your self as a unique a person, this will not have in reality befell to you in any manner." "You can't and must now not love some other person till you first decide to like yourself first because it all starts with you and within you."

These are not anything but simply a number of the shallowness tonics, worldviews, and directives we will supply to ourselves or sensible tips we get to indicate some methods via that can end up extra a success and thru which we can stay a life of fulfilment. There are also methods thru which we are able to find our strategies and paths to self-actualization.

Self-love is crucial to residing properly. It impacts picks and things you select for your self and your friends, the proper image you mission and constitute at domestic, spiritual circle, political circle, at your administrative center, and the way you address the problems in your life. It is therefore pertinent and especially necessary in your well being and improvement which you recognize the manner to control your existence, your courting, and your ambitions.

What is self-love? Is it one component you may be able to get via a beauty makeover or a logo-new set of garments? Can you get a variety of it through reading one thing that is inspirational? Or, will a logo-new relationship reasons you to love your self greater? The right reaction to those issues is not what you must be looking for but how you could end up better and enhance for your mental health. Even although they experience fantastic, happy and are notable, you can not grow in self-love till you do what is vital

Self-love is not simply genuinely feeling appropriate and clever. It is definitely a kingdom of appreciation and being inquisitive about one's fulfillment and for oneself. These feelings and emotions grow from actions that support our physical, psychological and different boom, and psychological development. Self-love is some thing that continues converting and constantly being tough to define or hold close. It is some thing that grows via actions that mature in us and also make us mature. When we act in approaches wherein amplify self-love us, we start to be given a good deal better our shortcomings and additionally our strengths and wonderful sides as something that can not be modified however need to be improved upon, continuously evaluated and consolidated. We do now not want to give an explanation for our weak spot for the subsequent character as she or he additionally has his or her personal. Doing so will amount to proscribing your self and increasing our character weaknesses when we do no longer absolutely ought to do so.

Prescription for Self-Love and Mental Health

1. Become mindful. People who've a whole lot of self-love have a tendency to grasp what they

anticipate, feel, and want. They are aware of the whole thing about themselves. More so they are positive human beings and feature positive vibe round them in any respect time and usually act on their strengths and weaknesses, rather than on what others want them to do or what the others assume from them.

2. You should act on what you want in place of on what you only want. You love yourself after you may draw back from one component that feels smart and thrilling to what you desire to stay robust, cantered, and moving forward on your life, instead. By staying focused on what you wish, you switch away from automatic behaviour patterns that get you into hassle, keep you stuck in the past, and lessen self-love.

three. Practice good self-care. You will love yourself loads after you are taking better care of your basic wants. People who're sincerely excessive in self-love and self belief always feed themselves with the right quantity of high quality energy every day through healthful activities, reasonable discussions, proper sleep, logical wondering, sound vitamins, exercise, intimacy, and healthy social interactions.

four. Set obstacles. You'll love your self a variety of after you set limits or say no to parent, love, or sports that exhaust or harm you bodily, emotionally and spiritually in all components, or express negatively who you are certainly really are.

five. Safeguard your self from hatred. Bring the right wide variety of useful human beings into your life each day. This is one manner via which you can improve your persona and make yourself higher. I love the time period 'frenemies'. This way pal and enemy at a time. It is a phrase that I found out from my neighbour who grew to become a very good pal or perhaps I ought to say who turned a family eventually. It describes and captures therefore well the idea of "friends" who typically take superb delight for your emotional disturbance, pain, mental shutdown, and loss in preference to to your happiness, winnings, achievements, and success. My notion to you here: Do away with such poisonous people in case you cannot change them! There is no sufficient time on your hand to retain that kind of humans to your lifestyles. You do now not have any time to waste on human beings that display to be parasitic in your existence. So, you want to run faraway from them. Let them see signs and symptoms that pretty says, "I certainly love my life and myself and want the nice for myself" When you do this, you will start to love and to appreciate your self an increasing number of, and you'll begin gaining the right attention that your life actually required.

6. Forgive your self of any wrongdoing and let burst off the beyond. Human beings, specially younger folks who are just growing, may be so difficult on themselves now and again. The bad components of being responsible for our deeds is punishing ourselves and being difficult on ourselves an excessive amount of for the mistakes we made in the past. You want to understand that your mistakes are a part of your studying method and developing phases. You should certainly accept your great (the incontrovertible reality which you're no longer best) earlier than you may be able to really love

your self. Practice being less arduous on yourself once you build a slip-up. Remember, there are no disasters if you have discovered and grown out of your mistakes; there are best instructions found out.

7. Live intentionally. You will accept and love your self a number of, anything is happening to your life when you stay with cause and layout. Your reason does no longer want to be crystal clean to you. If you need to degree a significant and healthful lifestyles, you ought to decide to make decisions and select the options that aid your purpose, and that you really experience true about your self whilst you achieve them. You have to discover a purpose to your life and need to paintings closer to reaching the ones purposes and realizing your dream. You will love yourself plenty in case you see yourself carrying out what you started out and aimed to acquire. For you to without difficulty do this, you ought to establish and verify your living intentions and long-term goals.

It is viable that you also emerge as extra conscious and self enough emotionally. Just consider what stage you need to move and how far you want to reach in existence. People will start appreciating you most effective when you exercising self-love and display unrestraint goals to reap your dreams. It is true that you just will totally love someone the most amount as you want yourself. If you show self-love that I am speakme approximately here, in a way that indicates passions and determinations, you will no longer best achieve your goals however at the equal time allow and inspire other individuals who are such as you to explicit themselves within the equal way. There is a lot of self-love that you have genuinely were given for yourself, and you want to begin displaying that for the arena to peer. The higher prepared and equipped you're for turning into a higher individual and geared up to make your courting grow the more healthy you come to be mentally and bodily. Even greater, you will start to draw in many like minds, situations, and occasions to you that help your properly-being. You need to display forth your mild and help make global a better location for anyone to stay.

Chapter 10: Believe In Yourself To Build A Business Empire

This bankruptcy has been designed to help you get the self-esteem, perception, and imaginative and prescient you need to succeed in any business. The bankruptcy is written with the marketers in thoughts. This is because many business proprietors, marketers and SME founders, start-united statesfold up within a short length because they cannot preserve up with the momentum. So this chapter is designed to assist them paintings on their enterprise and become higher at what they do.

At the stop of this bankruptcy, you are expected to apprehend why you should have the essential competencies, beliefs, esteem, and worldview which might be wished for a successful day out in each enterprise.

What distinguishes a hit commercial enterprise owners are so giant in this sort of manner that, though they can be explored but can not be exhausted in this book. They all have unique enterprise outlooks that contribute to their achievement, make their businesses outlive them, and live applicable for a completely long time. Their enterprise outlook is different from that of regular oldsters, and this is the primary thing that places them on the success music. That without a doubt manner that the recipe for achievement is thinking out of the container, being creative and modern in any such manner that you are capable of solve issues within the network. Therefore, it is not most effective essential however essential which you placed your wondering cap on usually if you are to become a wonderful entrepreneur.

In addition to that, whether as a start-up or pro enterprise owner who planned to diversify or move to every other business terrains that are completely extraordinary from the acquainted ones, you want to apprehend your enterprise surroundings, your situation, your temperament together with the circumstance of this new environment in which you locate your self. You should also make conscious efforts to improve the area of interest or commercial enterprise surroundings inside that you suppose you could be triumphant. What is also essential is that you ought to be prepared to effect changes inside the lives of humans and need to be prepared to proffer answers to the perennial issues that characterised your society or the world at large. Business approach fixing problems in imaginative methods and what is critical is the more trouble you remedy, the higher, rich and diagnosed you emerge as in the society. That way your fulfillment lies on your perception and outlook. It centres for your vanity and self belief.

When finding out your very own approach to the challenges of entrepreneurship, it's going to make your enterprise develop in soar if you can examine from the stories of others and leaders in your commercial enterprise.

Believing success should come without fighting for it's miles lethal mistake that it is easy to make as a commercial enterprise coach or an entrepreneur. Many naïve entrepreneurs, who are just appearing on the enterprise scene, accept as true with fulfillment should come at the primary trial, however this isn't always usually the case. There are one of a kind methods you could rent to make your commercial enterprise expand and tick, but you have to by no means take the shortcut to achievement. You need to also ensure that nothing tampers along with your self assurance or derail your vision.

Chapter 11: How To Develop Confidence In Order Not To Struggle With Failure

This bankruptcy is carefully designed which will learn how critical confidence on your non-public growth is. This chapter has additionally been written to show you how you can upturn that thought of failure that has been consistently making you doubt your electricity and capability. It is likewise designed to help you see the manner out of each problem you locate on your enterprise. At the cease of this bankruptcy, you ought to be capable of apprehend how to build your self assurance, how to radiate positivity and love. You should additionally be able to understand how crucial to the fulfillment of your commercial enterprise, logo and individual is confidence. To prevail, you ought to hold a positive level of self assurance. Furthermore, you should additionally be able to apprehend the way to eliminate each obstacle in your ways. You have to additionally be capable of recognize why suffering with failure does no longer worth some time and interest. So you are anticipated to examine on the way to awareness at the primary and cast off the trivial problems that may affect your mental health and self recognition.

A man with first rate confidence and corporation belief can move mountain even if the entire world doubts him so you have to care much less about what humans could say or what people are presently announcing in opposition to you. It isn't always simplest important but additionally necessary that you exude self assurance in all you do. You need to radiate self belief and advantageous vibes in case you need your enterprise to emerge as what you want. The following are approaches to broaden confidence in your self:

1.   Give Without Expecting Anything in Return: Although, at first, this may look like a daunting undertaking and very unreasonable, however if you are to succeed in any commercial enterprise, particularly enterprise inside the area of interest of the expertise economy, you have to be ready to give your excellent with out watching for whatever in go back from the humans. Many specialists, pupils

and a hit people in commercial enterprise had established that first rate opportunities and success should only come your manner whilst you start giving your great and including values to humans with out attaching any string to it. That way you ought to undertake an method in which you anticipate not anything from humans after you might have furnished them the satisfactory you can. One way is to regularly dole out ideas on a way to improve or set-up a business to many people with whom you might recollect enterprise companions or the ones you're inquisitive about their movements and efforts. You need to constantly do that with out soliciting for some thing in return. Let me tell you what is going to take place in case you keep with that exercise. In no time, you may be confident and plenty of human beings will look up to you. In addition to that you will begin getting extra than you could have requested from them or charged them. That might be because you usually deliver them your satisfactory which makes them be triumphant and come to be higher. This will improve your intellectual health and self belief and make you get higher in what you do. Also, whilst the ones people emerge as a hit and achieve their desires, it is simplest natural that they'll pay you back in triple folds, if not in economic it may be in different ways.

As an entrepreneur or emblem, this principle ought to be carried out on your enterprise in case you actually need to develop and be triumphant. As a startup, you have to focus on the offerings you're rendering and must be ready to offer your customers the great that you may offer.

2.   Keep Control of Your Vision: Jack Ma, the business multi-millionaire this is additionally known as the daddy of current dropshipping commercial enterprise in China, is the founder and guiding hand this is making Alibaba blossom on a day by day basis. Despite Alibaba great, money, achievement, etc. Alibaba's street to acceptance outdoor China become now not an smooth one. There had been collection of court cases regarding counterfeit or pretend matters offered-out on the positioning from one-of-a-kind quarters and that affected the enterprise in one manner or

every other. And, similarly to that, the hassle becomes exacerbated whilst Jack Ma tries to put his company as a site different groups use as a supply of wholesale products for the duration of the world. There became an inflow of people of low integrity who saw that as street to perform their nefarious activities. This should have discouraged Jack Ma, however no, he turned into no longer discouraged. He solid on and were given his project executed. Therefore you need to in no way lose awareness of your dream or vision. To increase your self assurance and positioned your business at the proper footing, even though you are facing some demanding situations at a point in time, you need to by no means discouraged. You ought to usually be of the opinion that you'll get any impediment in your manner. As an entrepreneur, I recognize once in a while trying to get your rhythm may be hard – trying to balance business with private issues might be irritating, however you have to by no means be discouraged. Therefore, when demanding situations come in your business, you need to in no way shirk your responsibility or shrink back out of your vision. You must decide to get your imaginative and prescient and goals carried out and must ensure that your desires and goals are carried out.

3.   Understand the Power of Good Name: Your idea is what many desires depend upon and so you want to turn that concept right into a logo. That isn't always possible until you get your mind fully charged and your self belief fully boosted. When you see yourself as a person who the complete world depends on, that concept of yours becomes something of a springboard so as to lead to profitable commercial enterprise for other human beings. Therefore you ought to make sure that your ideas are well packaged to the quantity that t turns into a family name. What this means is which you must have a larger photograph even though the modern scenario appears discouraging. You ought to also be geared up to set up your emblem from the begin. Anything which could have an effect on your emblem and reputation negatively must be speedy treated. You must additionally, as an entrepreneur, discover a manner to copyright, franchise and logo your enterprise in this sort of manner that

no person can take benefit of you or thieve your idea.

In this generation in which turning into one's personal boss is progressively turning into the order of the day, it's miles a known fact that the dream of entrepreneurship and also the realities of entrepreneurship commonly deliver a harsh reality that maximum start-up and enterprise owners aren't organized for. Most times, what they get isn't like what they expected or envisaged. However, will that suggest that an entrepreneur ought to now not pass forth as soon as the going gets hard and troubles start rearing their unpleasant heads?

Having commenced my entrepreneurial adventure in the past few years, I can't begin to spotlight the wide variety of instances that I were instructed (through others moreover as myself) that my marketing strategy can not workout and that my business plan will lead to my destruction, and that success is not positive and surprisingly unlikely. I accept as true with you may imagine how excruciating that might be, especially when you get rejected by means of folks who need to assist you to develop and grow to be higher. Now, I need you to assume how self-inflicted doubt, low vanity, fear of failure and failing to do something drastic for yourself ought to restriction your chance at greatness. I additionally experienced that, I struggled with failure until I realized that the social validation and people's approval I became looking for changed into no longer the issue I wanted. What I became locating changed into not wherein I turned into searching. The approval changed into within me and turned into deeply buried deep among in me. So I took as my next undertaking and sole duty to unearth the potentials I want.

Often as soon as one starts offevolved in this journey we generally tend to assume human beings close to us to be our largest and loudest supporters. This isn't always always the case and it from time to time makes us think that for the reason that human beings around us, or our network isn't approving our processes or organizations then we're failure. That is not proper. We need fantastic strength to propel us to new and greater huge heights and that rejection could be the component we really need every so often. Therefore do no longer war with failure however use the whole thing on your manner as a stepping stone for your greatness. Typically this could not be clean to do. Therefore you need to emerge as your biggest fan and loudest supporter. It is simplest whilst you begin to look inside yourself for the energy that you want that you may honestly achieve life.

In every business, similar to existence in general, it is not only essential but crucial that you bring yourself once there may be not anything or nobody to carry you or cheer you on. Always choose to ignore the negativity from any nook and every course. Instead, you ought to consciously decide to stoke your fireplace. You should additionally make certain which you fire from all cylinders in case you want to get the job done and get your business to the world level.

Furthermore, you should dig deep in order o unearth the treasure which you are seeking, word that worth and start to unearth it – at the start, it could be painful or exhausting, and you can even cry due to the ardour you have got for what you're doing. However while you are performed and sooner or later get your heart choice, you'll be grateful that you in no way cease. It is unwavering doggedness, resoluteness, and resolution that would be the wished muse in your boom and fulfillment of your business. Each individual to your corporation need to function a source of motivation for you. You ought to continually see them as motives for now not backing down in your profession or imaginative and prescient. As a small scale enterprise proprietor or entrepreneur or tutor, you ought to continuously see your clients and students as supply of motivation. You should see them as people that their success depends on you and for this reason you cannot have the funds for to backpedal or give up. There is an aphorism that asserts, "no price ever came easy," You need to constantly hold every door at fulfillment open. Therefore, you must begin a sequence of events that may lead a lot of humans to you, and that might open your doors to success. It method that each one you have got were given to do is to begin making matters fall in area. Never battle with failure or anticipate every person to help you prevail.

Chapter 12: How To Develop Public Speaking And Positive Mindset

This chapter has been cautiously designed that will help you broaden a wonderful and growth attitude. At the cease of this chapter you must be able to apprehend and highlight things that you could do if you want to boost your public speaking prowess, how you may shut out screw ups and awareness on fulfillment and, how you could discover your strong factors and construct on it in the sort of way which you becomes a better person in the society. This chapter is also designed to present you an insight into how you can own a boom mind-set as an individual and how you may improve your act as an entrepreneur. By studying this bankruptcy, you have to be capable of apprehend those things that can imbue your thoughts with positivity and at the equal time, assist your enterprise develop.

An person with a fixed mindset believes that his or her intelligence is static, while an individual with exceptional intellectual health and boom attitude believes and knows that his or her intelligence can nonetheless be advanced and advanced on. But later see probable likes to include demanding situations, directly react to his setbacks, and see setback and postpone as herbal paths to mastery of enterprise endeavours and life. The distinction among these extremes has notable implications for intellectual fitness, self cognizance, motivation, productivity, and confidence. When one desires success, pursue something more large in existence or is in pursuit of happiness, excessive degree of intellectual brings a high-quality attitude. It also ends in a excessive degree of self awareness that is the entirety which you need to succeed. This is the grasp key which could help one gain the desired desires. Mental fitness is synonymous with increase and kingdom of one's thoughts and consciousness in life.

A increase attitude or excessive level of intellectual health consists of a considerable effect on commercial enterprise effectiveness and might be a determinant of fulfillment in lifestyles. It is a important problem keeping apart high achieving college students from those who battle inside the faculties and it is also the best defining aspect that determines a a hit or failed commercial enterprise or idea. It is also the setting apart factors between a successful entrepreneur and a failed one. Mindset is so commonly noted in the context of its programs for commercial enterprise and education. A boom mindset has been again and again called a strong predictor of business or educational fulfillment. It commonly increases an entrepreneur or students' motivation, grades, accomplishment, and ratings. Also, a growth attitude is a sturdy pillar for fulfillment in business and every different human endeavour. Therefore in case you have to succeed in what you do you should own a attitude that is very adaptive to exchange and prepared to learn.

Public speaking will facilitate your increase, increase your business, solidify your community, foster your relationships, help you get new enterprise, and growth your online presence very quickly. However, growing confidence as some distance as business and tutoring are involved occasionally does no longer come certainly.

I never get concerned or idea approximately public talking until my life took a dramatic turn: I used to be a shy character who does now not want to ask query, speak or improve voice or bother to take price in any get together I found myself. But when it dawned on me that developing a unique persona and getting my character and self logo to where it may be visible to the complete world needs my energetic participation and contribution, I decided to study the artwork of public speakme. I began attempting to find new ways to get exposed, increase my base, improve on my network of buddies.

To put my life so as, I started out reading marketers who're a hit of their own proper. I targeted on those people in my niche and came to one accurate but honest conclusion: Successful humans are confident public audio system.

All my existence, earlier than I took price, I turned into not constantly snug speaking earlier than a big number of audiences. That become because I never believed I may be an awesome speaker. I used to be timid and shy all due to the fact I thought I become no longer reduce out for public talking.

Despite that, I even have in no way, for once, walked far from a task or shirked my obligation. Having found out early on that invisibility is a ways worse than failure, I placed my wondering cap on and started out locating solutions to my problems. Public talking had allowed me to push my profession to a new stage, granting get entry to to humans and places I by no means had before, and it had made me emerge as a person who usually thinks that turning into higher every day is the favor that I can do myself.

To be successful at what you do, you don't want to be a guru or a terrific rhetorician, but you must ensure you supply many memorable keynotes, schooling seminars and talks around the globe. As you try this, your enterprise will grow and also you becomes a higher man or woman amongst your peers

Public Speaking Creates Opportunities To State Your Feeling and Views

Public speakme leads to wealth. It will assist you in building your network of pals. It will also give you cult-like followership, foster your relationships, assist you land new contracts, grow your new commercial enterprise, get activity offers and growth your social media presence.

Most people do now not seem to be comfortable speaking earlier than a huge wide variety of audiences. According to numerous reports, approximately the two-third of the arena populace suffers from speech tension. Therefore, in case you currently belong to the organization of those people who are suffering speech anxiety, I need you to recognize that nothing is surely wrong with you (you are satisfactory and perfect the way you're) - it's miles a psychological nation that you can regulate and recover from with. I became as soon as for your shoe. Anytime I get in front of an audience or holding microphone or dealing with the digicam or charged to address greater than ten humans; I would emerge as worried and over-excited which on occasion would make me forget about what I changed into to inform the humans. I later overcame this through aware effort.

Here are a few cues for a superb mindset:

1. Have an Unrivaled Understanding of the Subject Matter

Ken Linder, a international-famend public speaker said, when you decide to discuss topics and troubles that you recognize, have sufficient know-how on and you are obsessed with, humans have a tendency to consider you and subsequently accept as true with your judgment on different matters as well. That actually approach that a speaker need to find a manner to apprehend the problem count number, preserve mastery and show that she knows than her target market to win them over. Confident audio system increase their enjoy by using understanding their difficulty depend in a way that mystifies and puzzles their target market. The works you are taking time to investigate are observed and appreciated by way of your teeming target market. That is due to the fact the genuineness comes forth thru the transport of your speech.

Avoid picking subjects which you don't have any passion. Trying to train a topic or enterprise, you have no strong passion for is a super way to spoil your attitude and vanity.

Confident public audio system deliver convincing arguments by riveting the numerous but applicable statistics in what they talk. They cite examples and give manageable cues. Therefore, you should be prepared.

Read, have a look at and memorize key concepts. Accumulate exciting records, memories, rates, and examples. These can provide you with a fantastic mind-set, and because of that, you'll have rich and attention-grabbing content to give to human beings that are looking as much as you.

2. Always be prepared on your sports:

My greatest motto in existence is, "Be prepared, and also you might be fortunate." One of the best manner to prepare your self is to practice for hours before a mirror or earlier than some decided on buddies who can determine your strengths and weaknesses and proffer answers. You also can do a get dressed practice session in an empty area this is much less distractive to enhance your confidence. You ought to additionally now not neglect the strength of your mind. By reciting the speech on your thoughts time and again again, you can fast get your confidence boosted.

three. Use innovative and picturesque sentence.

By using visuals like slides, graphs, diagram, percentile, films, pix, newspaper headlines, reports, and so on. You'll be able to speak much less and draw your target market's attention like a magnet. It is useful for redirecting strain and attention out of your actual delivery.

Shift the target market's cognizance from you to the content you want to get across to them

Even the foremost dynamic audio system use mental imagery to maintain the attention of their audience. If you want to succeed as a enterprise educate, you have to be prepared to inspire, inform, energize thoughts and, at the equal time entertain human beings listening to you with the aid of ensuring what you deliver is worth subscribing to on this knowledge-based totally financial system and information-based totally economic system that international is currently going through.

Your audience desires to use the content material being given for his or her personal advantage, so make new, dramatic and inspiring statements which can deliver your content convincingly.

You must constantly lace your speech and content with phrases that symbolize actions, and that may charge them to take over the commercial enterprise world and domain names.

For your intellectual health, the use of effective diction and appealing mental imagery ought to be some thing which you always do in case you want to set yourself other than the rest. Spend terrific quantity of time on sprucing your presentation. When you have got catchy slogans, watchword and taglines people will see you as being specific from the others on your niche and so one can ultimately make your business develop. Therefore, you should have a unique fashion, manner of doing talking, color code, logo and a emblem this is distinct from the relaxation.

4. Announce your entry with boldness

Having a nerve and doubt are two distinct matters which can elicit distinct responses in enterprise. Hesitation creates limitations however having wonderful nerves do away with them and make your enterprise jump.

Start your commercial enterprise on a high-quality be aware. That is critical due to the fact being ambitious makes you appear larger than existence. It additionally draws to you the vital energy that can make your enterprise survive — your attitude, in addition to the way you start your business, is fairly important to the charge at which your commercial enterprise will develop. Therefore, in case you need your enterprise to experience astronomical boom, you have to be constructed on credibility and accept as true with.

five. Be Open to Feedback

Both effective and remarks will improve your self belief and make your enterprise develop in a way which you in no way imagined. Therefore you need to establish a channel thru which you could quickly talk and acquire remarks out of your patron. One aspect that could without difficulty assist a logo, be it small or massive usiness develop is review and comments. Therefore, you have to continually have it behind your thoughts that on your business, your clients need to actively take part. You need to design your enterprise in one of these way that the comments out of your customers may be used to create novel thoughts, design new merchandise, improve the great of your product, fulfill your customers, and supply your customers what they truely choice or offer custom designed products for your customers.

Although getting comments from your people can be uncomfortable and hurtful on occasion, however you must apprehend that the people who assess you are being real with you and the people that deal with you are the number one source via which your personality or logo may be assessed. That is due to the fact your friends and households won't want to hurt you with the reality. Therefore, you should now not completely rely upon them for the complete assessment of your performance. Any judgment and feedback on your commercial enterprise overall performance and private overall performance need to be used to push yourself harder and must be used to regulate your shortcomings and imperfection. You need to enhance with every review, remark, and comments because this is the simplest manner via which you could certainly enhance yourself and upgrade your mental health to be able to grow to be self aware and keep best intellectual fitness.

Chapter 13: Youth Mental Health 1.1 An Intersectionality Approach To Youth's Mental Health

The lives of contemporary youth are impacted by means of intersecting members of the family of energy that have an effect on their social, political, and financial participation, as well as their health and well being. Childhood consists of various populations which have visible a variety of lived stories and lifestyles chances. Recent statistics recommend that young human beings constitute 1/2 of the overall global population (Youth forum). Of these teenagers, one fourth (or 1.8 billion) is between the a while of 15 and 29 (Global Youth Development Index, 2016When children are supplied with the possibility, peace, safety, gender fairness, and get entry to to primary wishes. They emerge as the force in the back of destiny development. However, funding in youngsters requires equitable get right of entry to to training, meaningful employment, financial increase, and inclusive and supportive environments in which they can thrive. Despite this, global children poverty has reached alarming ranges, even as get right of entry to to activity security, schooling, and capabilities alternate is diminishing. The social exclusion of youngsters is plenty higher amongst immigrant and radicalized teens and people handling a bodily disability or mental health demanding situations. Besides the intersection of age, gender, race, elegance, sexual orientation, a lack of systemic intervention and prevention services, children can enjoy abuse, stigma, and all varieties of violence, consisting of sexual violence. Youth sexual violation takes place inside their homes, groups, and society at huge, both at some point of peace and war, at some point of their displacement or migration, and even at the same time as dwelling in a safe surroundings.

The dimensions of stigma, sexual violation, and sexual orientation amongst youth increase vulnerabilities, worry, and the prevalence of mental fitness situations. The 2016 World Health Organization (WHO) report observes that 20% of the arena's kids and youth be afflicted by some shape of intellectual health situation. Studies propose that today's adolescents's mental health is encouraged some distance greater by means of social than biomedical factors. The era of modern-day children is likewise left with a lot unmet health and intellectual health needs due to the shortage of institutional capacity, sustainable funding, and inclusion of adolescents voices in decision-making tactics. These elements can negatively impact their present and threaten their destiny as they transition from youth to maturity.

This series asserts that teenagers's human rights matters and that their voices, lived conditions, hopes, and dreams, and resilience should no longer be disregarded. This belief introduced together the 3 editors of this ebook—each from a one-of-a-kind field of know-how—and a collection of dedicated pupils, network participants, and teenagers from around the world and interdisciplinary backgrounds.

The chapters in this e book present quite a number perspectives on kids and intellectual fitness. The intersectionality framework informs the overarching theoretical perspective. This framework pushes modern-day young people intellectual fitness discourse past the micro-level or individualized care model to task complex and interlocking systems of strength, privilege, and oppression on the neighborhood and transnational degrees. The scholarly contributions right here stem from various disciplines aiming to confront the ones micro family members that could undermine adolescents's intellectual fitness while grounding the discourse historically and materially. It extends from adolescence's lived experiences to encompass social environments, economic and political participation, and destiny opportunity. Contributors examined those elements that bring about youth's displacement or entrapment, considering how they're constructed into various social and criminal categories as migrants, refugees, illegalized folks, immigrants. Citizens are may be first-generation, intergeneration, or a couple of generations. Other socially built identities, consisting of local location, gender, race, class, sexual orientation, appearance, own family family members and own family repute, and physical fitness and mental fitness, are in addition explored. The authors unpack how these conditions growth adolescents vulnerabilities to violence and stigma or circumscribe their inclusion and exclusion in their homes, faculties, and groups.

WHO considers mental fitness challenges are to be preconditions for different sorts of intentional and accidental illnesses and accidents. Few sources are available to adolescents in need of mental fitness guide. In addition to this, a sequence of things— structural inequities, conflict, poverty, racialization, discrimination, gender violence, bullying, and stigma—may additionally often prevent them from gaining access to those assets. Moreover, those same elements regularly similarly violate the human rights and livelihood of affected kids. On the floor, the kids's intellectual fitness may also look like "micro issues." Still, it's miles associated with a sequence of conditions that require a tackling of chronic root causes and a surmounting of each nearby and global obstacles. However, today's adolescents isn't always a passive populace. Despite increasing challenges, teenagers are often the force in the back of campaigns and social moves, building desire for a higher destiny. Their political engagement and leadership are also directed at tackling troubles that have an effect on them in my opinion and their environment and transnational groups as they intersect with each other. While we must have a good time modern-day young people's resilience, we are able to pause, listen to their voices, and study from their reports; this will enable us to work in the direction of a teens-centered international network.

Health is formed via more than one fluids and bendy, socially constructed categories of race/ethnicity, gender, age, social magnificence, and migrant status that intersect and impact micro and macro-structural degrees. An intersectional approach requires researchers to collect records approximately how humans live their lives and account for the numerous affects that shape those lives. Intersectionality can be visible as explaining structures of domination and subordination which can be interactive and create complicated intersections resulting in a kingdom of 'trans-identity' experienced at the individual, structural and coverage stages. An intersectional-kind evaluation locations the importance of strength and its position in developing and perpetuating discrimination and oppression fundamental when considering the issue at hand. Our overview's intersectional analysis located that more than one axes of social classes motivated migrant youngsters intellectual fitness at a personal degree, school level, and structural level. Adjusting to a new college device changed into a disturbing experience for immigrant and refugee kids. Many confronted stereotyping and labeling incidences inclusive of being called 'refugee' or 'silly.' The assemble of 'refugee' changed into related to negative assumptions about the youths' ability and stigmatized vulnerabilities (such as belonging to the lowest earnings quintile) in place of focusing on their strengths. The labeling disempowered teens and undermined their self-confidence and relationships of agree with. Cultural war, social rejection, perceptions of discrimination, and marginalization contributed to emotions of lack of confidence for kids and ended in bad instructional performance and a decline in intellectual health. Our findings validate in advance findings on the perception of discrimination at faculty or neighborhood and its destructive effects on migrant youngsters's sense of belonging.

Supportive environments (schools, communities, and neighborhoods) and healthful relationships (family and friends) facilitate health, corporation, and empowerment. Multiple intersecting axes were operating at the faculty stage affected kids powerfully. Generally, faculties performed a dual role; to start with, they have been areas wherein migrant children felt insecure, marginalized, intimidated, and stressed, however as the feel of belonging to the faculty or 'college connectedness' grew, it lessened the settlement stress, and schools have become heavens in cover. As migrant teens obtained fluency inside the English language and familiarized themselves with the dominant society way of life, their friends became more accepting of them. Schools are essential places to analyze; they're spaces where migrant youngsters health and social needs can be identified and addressed. The preference to belong to the dominant society and not abandon their ethnic identification placed adolescents in acculturative pressure. Immigrant and refugee youth's terrible encounters with intersecting types of racism and discrimination have been primarily based on their race, seen look, and apparel. These encounters impacted the kids's feel of belonging and expression of cultural identities. By 'silencing their selves,' adolescents kept away from expressing themselves or disclosing their ethnic identification. This coping mechanism helped them keep away from embarrassment and hurting their shallowness. The migrant kids have been an increasing number of privy to their mother and father' challenges and struggles about instructional and professional qualifications no longer being recognized, deskilling unemployment, and underemployment. The infant regarded themselves in their households' context and found out that their families confronted amazing economic hardships. It is known that radicalized Canadians stumble upon persistent blocks from the first-class paying jobs the country has to offer and feature three instances higher poverty charges than non-radicalized households.

Working situations for newly settled people and families have deteriorated with the decline in core federal investment. Withdrawal of national authorities duties (federal devolution) from offering agreement offerings and cutbacks on immigrant service organizations has disabled specialized carrier provision, circle of relatives counseling, and mental fitness services for ethnic-racial businesses.

1.2 Precarious Status

You begin to have breakdowns, unpleasant matters that overwhelm you at the internal. It makes it difficult to respire, and the room spins. You sob to sleep via these hard moments. You scrape your hands until there are purple traces and sit down there for hours. You suck into your thumb's inner flesh. All the same, you preserve as nevertheless as you could. When your mom is snoozing, crying becomes a habit of doing when in mattress. You fake the entirety is ok in the course of the day, that the scratches are due to a few bizarre rash, and that nightmares cause your sleepless nights.

— 21-year-old adolescents dwelling in Canada with precarious popularity because 2011

When thinking about the connection among immigration status and intellectual fitness amongst migrant kids in Canada, precariousness affects are pervasive and widespread. Inherent to the definition of precocity are poignant implications for establishing a sustained sense of protection, safety, and predictability—the relevance of well-mounted intellectual fitness and health—the nuanced courting among immigration reputation and precocity reviews migrant. Youth bureaucracy Canadian society's participation and get entry to and underpins the internalization of the alienation, disempowerment, and shortage of protection created with the aid of the illegalization of the non-popularity body. While linkages among mental fitness and precarious immigration status are emergent in the academic literature, scholarly paintings around this effective and chilling intersection is enormously scarce. The literature is further constrained while considering the Canadian context and truely absent while narrowed in scope to the youth demographic. This bankruptcy seeks to explain a few primary mechanisms by which precocity trauma influences the migrant toddler's intellectual health and brings interest to the pressing need for meaningful intervention at the scientific, network, and coverage levels.

We adopt this work as Canadian-born the front-line youngsters employees situated at community-based totally organizations in downtown Toronto, striving to negotiate our complex relationships with electricity and privilege in constructing significant alliances with precarious migrant youngsters. Much of what's unpacked in this chapter attracts upon our front-line paintings and network-based totally studies with youngsters who've courageously shared their each day grappling with the impact of immigration guidelines on their get right of entry to to critical offerings, relationships, and their internal worlds. These colourful, various, and all too regularly excluded voices that this chapter strives to enlarge. Our overarching intention is to accomplish that with integrity, transparency, and cohesion, mapping out a theoretical framework grounded in a trauma-knowledgeable, anti-oppressive, and intersectional technique. We are trying to find to renowned the nuance and diversity of identity, each our own and those of the kids we work with, and to invoke feminist praxis to meaningfully empower and engage younger people while assembly them. Our work is deeply rooted inside the reputation that precarious migrant adolescents revel in more than one interlocking forms of oppression, which happen each in phrases of heightened vulnerability to interpersonal violence, as well as structural situations that feature to shape get entry to to power, resources, and safety. Therefore, interventions are required at the person degree and need to have interaction with and deal with the insidious systemic inequities that impact migrant kids's intellectual fitness and contribute to complex and often intergenerational histories of trauma.

Despite their interwoven relationship, discourses round immigration popularity and mental fitness are frequently relegated to 2 distinct rules and praxis our bodies. This illusory disconnect fails to capture the lived truth of precocity. Particularly for children at important developmental durations of their lives and similarly invisibilizes the urgent want for action. We argue that to efficaciously co-believe collaborative, empowered, and meaningful options to addressing migrant young people's intellectual fitness want accelerated interest and tenderness around this nuanced intersection is required. Indeed, notwithstanding representing an arguably developing populace in Canada, the invisibility of the precarious migrant teens revel in is awesome in its digital omission from all dominant discourse ranges, together with educational literature and network-based supports the attention of the general populace. Such pervasive marginalization influences are complicated and intersect in many ways with different markers of identity along with race, age, language, gender, and sexuality, to provide multilayered limitations to tremendous mental health effects for this populace.

Moreover, the inaccessibility of protected immigration popularity in Canada can exacerbate past demanding stories, further underlining the significance of nuanced, intersectional evaluation.

When thinking about young people's lived studies, it is important to notice that under their age, younger humans are much less probable than adults to have chosen to relocate to Canada in their very own volition. Many of the teenagers we paintings with survive extreme violence of their nations of starting place, the affects of which can be frequently exponentially compounded as soon as in Canada via challenges related to forced/ coerced migration, exile, and exclusion. And but, teens dwelling in Toronto, with an immigration popularity characterized by using the very precocity so implicated in intellectual health issues, are hardly ever afforded get right of entry to to relevant assist and continue to be mechanically denied essential offerings. Indeed, kids with precarious immigration fame can be considered disproportionately impacted by more than one interlocking structures of oppression, consisting of poverty and racism, due to their enormous exclusion from programming designed to combat such forces.

This chapter has been advanced in close collaboration with a neighborhood collective of teens residing with precarious immigration fame, such as community consultation within the shape of one-on-one interviews, recognition corporations, and the protected youngsters responses. We regret that contributors can't be credited through call for his or her contributions because of their identities' illegalization.

Participants have been invited for a focused group across the subject matter in query became prolonged to all participants of a Toronto-based newcomer adolescents group. Ten adolescents elected to participate and approved the audio recording of the 98-minute consultation. Three next one-on-one interviews have been carried out with folks that were not able to wait the focal point organization. All contributors had pre-present relationships with one or each people thru our paintings at our respective and often taking part, community-based totally agencies—a thing of observe in that it facilitated participation around a topic regularly fraught with fear, mistrust, and secrecy. As such, this awareness institution was informal and performed in the context of our set up community-based relationships rather than an educational organization. We maintained adherence to our organizational policies and the Ontario College of Social Workers and Social Service Workers code of ethics, shaping our purpose for safe and conscientious participation at some point of the records amassing method. Participants have been confident of confidentiality and in their proper to withdraw from the point of interest institution at any time. Individual guide changed into made available to teenagers ought to their involvement cause overwhelming or otherwise tough emotional stories.

These 13 primary informants represented ten countries of beginning, and 5 exceptional immigration statuses, which includes refugee claimants waiting for hearings, failed claimants present process the enchantment technique, global college students, Humanitarian and Compassionate applicants, and people with out a popularity at all. While this bankruptcy seeks to elevate collective attention around young people experiences of precarious immigration repute through the lens of intellectual health, there exists a intensity and breadth of complexities that enlarge nicely beyond the scope of our exploration. Therefore, future studies tips encompass a nuanced evaluation of different intersecting markers of identity, which includes sexuality and gender identity, race, u . S . A . Of beginning, language, and pre-migration reviews. Grounded in the voices of migrant kids, all of whom have lived experience navigating mental health challenges, discourse, and services even as keeping a precarious immigration reputation, the following number one issues emerged from our research: illegalization, get admission to and exclusion, identification formation, and uncertainty approximately the future. We do not forget those thematic groupings neither absolute nor exhaustive; as an alternative, we posit that they offer valuable inroads into a paradigm with the aid of which mental health and immigration coverage domain names be humanized, problematized, and taken into consideration in complex and nuanced relationships with each other.

1.3 Dancing Bodies, Spirits Soaring

Impacts of pedophilia inflicted on Afghan boys in Afghanistan on mental fitness:

Sexual violation is a kind of pederasty, and in music, arts and crafts, oral history, and literature, a homoerotic and pedophilic association with boys have ancient origins and strains. Boys and girls had been concern to maiming and mutilation in ancient cultures and had been used in the Renaissance and well into the eighteenth century for photo sexual activities, such as pornography. Pederasty and homoerotic affairs with teenagers, however, emerged as social conventions at numerous points in history and in one of a kind components of the sector, on the only hand, but on the opposite, they have been denounced or suppressed. The definition of 'childhood' and the 1989 United Nations Convention on the Rights of the Child, two critical discourses, have modified our belief of those relationships from embracing them as social conventions to seeing them as deviant and pedophilic acts. Today, numerous states have followed institutional law, guidelines, and strategies that, at the same time as assisting victims and their households, deter, discourage, and area sexual offenders. Despite this, interior their families, training, and cultures, and with the aid of friends, outsiders, or others in positions of authority, boys seem to fall victim to human smugglers, sex site visitors, and pedophiles. In 2016 by myself, over seventy three million boys witnessed a few form of sexual violation, consistent with a United Nations (UN) survey. As UN Special Representative Zainab Hawa Bangura determined, boys in war zones are becoming extra at risk of sexual violence. They face most important outcomes, consisting of sexually transmitted ailments, bodily injury, and depression, and psychological distress. In Afghanistan, boys' sexual violation is called the "Bacha (boy) Bazi (play)" exercise. While the influence of armed conflict on Afghan faculty-age youngsters and teens in Afghanistan has been documented in current years, little is thought approximately the consequences of sexual violation on mental health. Sex and sexuality are framed as private constructs, and public shaming and disgrace may be introduced on by means of conversations approximately sexual violations. By drawing on anti-colonial and analytical feminist research, this chapter incorporates secondary proof and the writers' expert views working with Afghan populations in Afghanistan and Canada. Hence, the emphasis of this chapter is threefold. Second, it explores how a long time of conflict and militarised abuse have intensified Afghan boys' susceptibility (from 7 to 18 years of age) to stumble upon sexual violation. This bankruptcy ambitions to unpack the rejection or minimization of the word "Bacha Bazi" (playful act) via historicizing the controversy to task any sexual violation as a pedophile act. Bacha Bazi is a pedophilic act committed via guys against small boys in this chapter. We contend that the subculture of Dancing Boys or "Bazaar" is an extension of such an act through cloth and sexual ownership, colonial authority, and militarised misogyny. Third, we talk the possible intellectual fitness outcomes on Afghan boys of sexual violations inflicted by way of guys. Sexual violence may have a protracted-lasting have an impact on on boys as they can go through special kinds of trauma that could bog down their development, livelihood, potentialities, and possibilities for existence. We declare that the enforced feminization of Dancing Boys, or "Bazaar," wherein boys are uncovered to homoerotic gazes, bodily and sexual violence, public humiliation, and shame, will make contributions to pre-present mental health problems extra levels of trauma. Despite all adversities, although, it's miles crucial to word that Afghans have important stamina in recent a long time to confront boys' sexual abuse and provoke socio-political exchange. The most critical work is "The Kite Racer," which contributed to the lifestyle of "Bacha Bazi" being globally exposed. This was observed via a protest led by way of independent human rights businesses.

Commissions and social justice activists lift the veil of silence, each regionally and internationally, and problematize the debate on human rights and sexual violations. The Government of Afghanistan has given that developed a National Study on Bacha Bazi in Afghanistan, criminalizing pedophilia, sodomy, and homoerotic relationships among grownup guys and boys. However, sexual harassment among boys is rising because of corruption, and the absence of systemic motion to put into effect the rules. Culturally, until maturity at age 18, Afghans check with Afghanistan as male kids as "Bacha" or "boys" We also use the phrase "boys" in this bankruptcy to refer to this age range (ages 7-18).

Addressing the outcomes of pedophilia on mental fitness

For researchers and mental health experts to observe and stigmatize the controversy, the first step in investigating the intellectual fitness outcomes of sexual harassment inflicted on Afghan boys is to look at and stigmatize the discussion. Panter changed into told by means of their Afghan educational advisory panel to keep away from concerns about "rape" in their comparative evaluation of faculty-elderly kids as this became deemed culturally insensitive. This supports Ullah's declare that intercourse and sexual crime are considered in place of the sexual predator as dishonoring the sufferer and kinfolk. Therefore, this stigmatization can perpetuate the prevalence of sexual violation and prevent any talk, even therapy, about the possible mental health implications. Collectively, Afghan boys face overt and oblique abuse and militarised trauma experienced during their lifespans in opposition to their human rights. Child survivors of violent conflict must deal with common worrying lifestyles experiences from family and community loss, as Catani, Schauer, and Neuner cautioned, leading to the lack of necessities and harm to their social existence, ordinary lives, and training. Ninety percent of the three hundred faculty-aged children interviewed in Kabul are confirmed to have seen useless bodies or frame elements, eighty percentage of whom have established emotions of grief, tension, or failure to deal with their ordinary activities.

Continued abuse and extended social demanding situations offer volatile and continual stress for boys, impeding their improvement and strong increase even after the actual violence has ended. A wealthy tradition that considers children the coronary heart of the own family and boys a pillar of the network is left with a technology of boys born and raised in conflict with little danger to experience their youth. In truth, they suffer from warfare-related injuries bodily and psychologically, sexual abuse, and loss, among different adversities. Their conditions have compelled a few to take at the role of company and protector in their households once they require safety, specially after they have interaction in self-harm behaviors to address their plights and losses. The Afghan government identifies mental health as a first-rate fitness hassle going through Afghans but offers little or no guide offerings. The mental fitness impact of the sexual violation on boys is tough to degree because of disgrace and stigma and male gender roles that force boys to be discreet about their studies. While individuals react to their violations in a different way, extended violence might also purpose comorbidity or accentuate pre-existing mental health conditions or signs. However, intellectual health guide isn't always included with the aid of the number one fitness care machine in individual and collective trauma. The diversion of international aid assets is in part geared in the direction of increasing administrative center security for workers and brief education applications for healthcare companies. The World Bank's

Human Development Network reported in 2011 that there have been, on the time, simplest across the world recognized psychiatrists inside the usa, neither of whom practiced, and that there had been no educated clinical psychologists or psychiatric nurses inside the usa.

Traditionally, many Afghans cope with their mental health-associated issues through approaching family contributors or through prayer or reliance on religious leaders and traditional healers for remedy. Mental fitness issues are concept to be caused by awful spirits or "Jinns," witchcraft, or the evil eye, which must be pushed away thru marriage or 40-day treatments of herbs and restricted diets. In maximum cases, families take their cherished ones to traditional recuperation centers and shrines placed in rural regions with little resources in which people are chained to partitions or bushes.

However, a long time of battle and violence have even constrained traditional recuperation facilities' assets or disrupted their excellent of treatment. Hospitals' constrained mental fitness clinics follow the traditional model of care, with personnel receiving minimum put up-disturbing strain disorder (PTSD) enjoy. In widespread, responses by way of the authorities, network members, and intellectual fitness practitioners to people handling intellectual health challenges simplest serve to spotlight the overarching stigma attached to the discourse. Therefore, stigmatization serves as a barrier to sharing experiences of sexual violation or in search of or receiving intellectual health remedy. This cultural stigma similarly helps cultural relativism and the reluctance of western governments or even the United Nations Security Council (UNSC) to recollect boys' sexual violation as a be counted of human rights difficulty requiring worldwide intervention. The International Commission for Intervention in State Sovereignty has made provisions that after the host government fails to protect its population and does not take any measures to prevent violence against its children, a 3rd us of a may additionally interfere. The US and coalition troops have unnoticed the problem for many years, and the USA has kept away from the sexual violation of boys and rape by means of defining or limiting rape to girls and girls.

International corporations, including the UN and NGOs, have controlled to provide some advert hoc hospital therapy in Afghanistan. Their intellectual health programs are generally geared closer to decreasing strain via video games, sports, and humanities. This embodies a disconnect between the scientific potential and the mental fitness needs of Afghan human beings dealing with multilayered trauma in popular, and, in this situation, of Afghan boys who've experienced sexual violation. The intellectual health impact of the sexual violation on boys is complicated, directly affecting them and their families, groups, and the bigger society. For instance, boys discover themselves with out a alternative however to obey their proprietors and "lords" bodily, emotionally, and sexually. As a result, they expand complex codependent relations as a part of which the boy's oppression enables set up commodity strength. At the same time, the boy's safety and survival rest on the mercy of his owner. This consequences in feelings of entrapment, worthlessness, powerlessness, shame, and guilt. Studies on male survivors of sexual abuse display melancholy, low self-esteem, and tension, among other bodily, sexual, and mental fitness demanding situations.

While it is essential to provide expert intellectual health offerings to victims, it is equally important to well known the distinctive situations that divulge boys to abuse and people' coping mechanisms and resilience. For example, in war zones, children and children are confronted with clusters of adversities at the man or woman, family, network, and structural ranges. As such, addressing their mental fitness needs must go beyond the use of conventional signs of PTSD and observe broader units of predictors and outcome variables. In Afghanistan, where mental fitness demanding situations are an understudied discourse or silenced and addressed historically, remedy may be gradual and long term. Healing is excellent approached in the context of an individual's comfort zone. Since Afghans generally tend to accept as true with in conventional sorts of remedy, mental fitness specialists' offerings are better offered in cohesion with traditional healers. Together, they could heal for exchange to stigmatize remedy.

1.Four When Youth Get Mad Through a Critical Course on Mental Health

Mad is a political, reclaimed term used by people who have mental distress, disconnection, diagnosis, and remedy. The Mad Movement is an global political entity composed of those who self-become aware of as Mad and those who might also become aware of as patients, customers, survivors, and clients of the intellectual fitness machine seeking better care, support, and recognition. Growing out of this motion, Mad Studies has become an academic area of scholarship that seeks options to biomedical processes to "intellectual health" with the aid of centering the know-how, enjoy, analysis, and voice of the Mad, the affected person, customer, survivor, client, refuses, and user of the mental fitness gadget. In this, Mad Studies seeks to foreground Mad people's tales, expertise, and lived realities. It problems taken for- granted tactics to competence, purpose, common sense, and binaries of "well" and "unwell." It celebrates collective narratives and pushes for "sufferers" as researchers. It is altogether an unsettling of widespread techniques to ontology and epistemology. In addition, to do Mad paintings can be to purposely upset the dominant procedure of the research article, including the usage of the so-called goal and passive voice, foregrounding of evidence-based totally literature, and the "preferred"

165

presentation of findings. It follows that this chapter does the identical, for this isn't a studies article or evaluative report on an intervention. It is not a theoretical piece that seeks to tease out an ontological loophole or a methodological message on a particular epistemological predicament. Instead, it's miles a Mad narrative written with the aid of Mad humans approximately a Mad-informed path correlated with Mad-identified people for teens/young person social paintings college students who have been in general elderly 19–29. This piece seeks to emote rather than continue to be remote. It seeks to problematize as opposed to randomize, and it seeks no longer to create "proof" however to create connection and opportunity for individuals who can be curious approximately the equal. As is regularly the case in Mad work, this chapter starts with and centers the private.

What Do I Know About Youth and Mental Health?

Shortly after my own family moved to Canada, I have a awesome reminiscence of pacing my room, crying my eyes out approximately the warfare. With no earlier revel in of armed war (unlike my dad and mom), I felt loss and pain move thru my frame as if the conflict become unfolding proper there after which in Montreal. I turned into nine years antique. Each 12 months the depth of my emotions grew, about everything, real and imagined. As a teenager, I felt deeply with human beings; I felt with nature and inanimate gadgets. I additionally felt anger and would direct it at those who did me incorrect, people who bullied me, or even the ones close. I couldn't calm myself down. I could not find peace, except whilst consuming secretly after which restricting meals publicly. I lied approximately all of it-to cover the ache, the anger, the reality wherein I lived, and the ingesting. I lied about it to keep away from scrutiny, retribution, and loneliness.

High school was like this, and then I moved away to college. There, I changed into left to my very own gadgets, and the practices of self-damage took root. The leap forward came at a peer support group held at a girls's center in addition to volunteering on a crisis line. It additionally came from what journalist Jan has known as the "geographical remedy" from further training, from many long years of counseling and supports of all kinds.

Now, looking again on my childhood and teenagers, I marvel what could have took place if we had now not moved to Canada when we did. What turned into going to do if my mother and father had referred to as the authorities, if I had now not been capable of carry out academically, or if they had divorced? I could have confronted a lot more precocity if one/both of them had died or if we had lived in more poverty or threat. It might have been a whole exclusive sort of mental misery revel in if I had come out or been trans and could not make new pals. It would additionally have been an entire other revel in if I had faced racism each day. I became included by way of whiteness and dwelling in a white supremacist society, with all of the unearned privileges and passes that include being in this white is a gendered frame. These a great deal extra complex eventualities are not unusual ordinary experiences for children inside the lessons I educate on social work exercise, research, theory, and mental health and insanity procedures. There is an excessive amount of being carried out to the scholars no longer to react, experience, barrel among states, and be in ache and misery. I am taking into account the pupil who has had electroconvulsive therapy ("surprise") those last few months, of all the ones experiencing Islam phobia and Anti-Black Racism on their manner to class, and the scholars who're parenting by myself.

How do parents make it to class? How do they make ends meet? How do they cope with their pressure and distress from the outcomes of racism, cissexism, classism, ageism, and heterosexism? How do any of these students maintain going?

Main Body Youth Mental Health

Adolescence (ages 10–19) and emerging adulthood (a while 18–29) are considered the peak durations for intellectual unwell-health onset, with 75% of all person diagnoses beginning earlier than 25 years. At least one in 4 to five youth (a long time 15–24) will revel in mental distress and unwell-health in any given year, and on most university campuses, the rates of mental distress are growing every 12 months. Responses to this form of misery are usually dominated by means of psychiatry, psychology, nursing, social work, and different expert problematization paradigms. The mounted healing exercise is to invite questions via exam if you want to perceive the problems, diagnose, and treat the problems. When it involves adolescents, there is an more and more lengthy listing of issues to deal with.

In Canada, those issues include severe mental misery and sociality in

Aboriginal teens, trauma, discrimination, and absence of equitable get entry to to fitness take care of immigrant and refugee teens, substance use, and tension for a child who isn't always heterosexual, and the world over, "negative assist-looking for and engagement by young human beings in mental fitness offerings." Accordingly, calls had been made to consciousness greater sources, studies, and attention on children mental health. Indeed, the new Youth Mental Health Movement maintains to gain momentum, and an International Declaration on Youth Mental Health has been launched in Europe and around the globe. Intriguingly, the statement calls for a fundamental shift in thinking about and responding to teenagers's intellectual health desires that consist of fewer "paternalistic," expert services and extra children-led options that create wide systemic exchange. However, given the historical reliance on "paternalistic" diagnosis and remedy, it follows that young people/teenagers in my lecture rooms have been recognized with despair, tension, ADHD, bipolar disease, borderline personality sickness, and schizophrenia. As they observe inside and outside of class, they are taking medicinal drugs, being "treated" in hospitals, as well as taking part in professionally led organizations, counseling, and others help where and while they may be capable/accessible or safe. Such strategies of exam and "remedy" may additionally start early at "college," in which students who are not white, middle class, or docile are assessed as "behavioral," complex, disabled, or tough. Guardians are referred to as, faculty social people are concerned, and case notes grow. Students may be eliminated from "normal" classrooms as part of this process, may be removed from homes, and regularly handled with medicine. As files develop, so do drop-out rates, disconnection, and visits to hospitals and professionals. Sometimes, the treatments paintings for some time, however 3/four times, they do now not, and with out alternatives, the teachers, young people, and parents begin the cycle again. For revitalized children, those cycles can lead to apprehension and jail. These cycles can lead to more and more high rates of "schizophrenia" prognosis—experience, as mentioned earlier, of mental misery and all that has transpired for black children. Since I am part of a movement that sees the mental health device as full of right intentions and a excessive opportunity of iatrogenic injury, it is not that I am absolutely against analysis and "remedy" or scientific version techniques to "intellectual health," for I see the opportunities of strategic analysis to secure help or incapacity aid, for example. I also know what it is to be so very desperate to have a "box," a prognosis, and a plan from which to work for protection and safety.

However, like the ones who have declared the global need for a fundamental reconsider round youth intellectual fitness, I am extra interested in making room for and perpetuating a distinctive kind of communication. This communication sits underneath the umbrella of the research, writing, and radicalism known as critical intellectual health.

Critical Approaches to Mental Health

By crucial, I am citing qualitative pupil Corinne Glens. According to her, to be crucial is to carry to the middle that which is bigoted or inequitable or has blocked participation. It is to be interested, as Foucault turned into, in subjugated information or information that has been pushed aside and altogether disqualified by way of dominant or set up discourses. For example, Indigenous portions of information were/are totally disqualified by settler colonialism on this u . S .. Mass disqualification has taken region through the regulation, thru residential education. Through identification theft pressured sterilization, electroconvulsive remedy. The theft of land and useful resource befell through the criminalization of dissent and ceremony, some avenues. No psychiatric varieties of understanding about "intellectual health" were disqualified too. Kept on the margins of what counts as a "proper" or "rational" technique to mental well-being, this disqualification consists of conventional Chinese medicinal drug. (TCM), recuperation practices, including reeking and meditation, body, political, protest, and anti-poverty paintings. Only whilst the dominant subject/technique/discourse begins to "approve"/permit/benefit from the opportunity approach/discourse that inroads are made (in addition to co-options). It is "expertise fascism" whilst most effective the clinical/clinical technique to mental fitness is widely known. So we're left with options to psychiatry which might be few and some distance between, or inaccessible, "dubious," or scientifically unsanctioned.

Most importantly, we're left with alternatives to psychiatry that are not often as lower priced in Canada as psychiatric strategies of exam, incarceration, seclusion, medicinal drug, intervention, and evaluation. Are we Mad to push for extra, ask for more for ourselves, our youth, and how we train notions of care and compassion? I assume not.

Chapter 14: Youth Mental Illness

Adolescent temper problems encompass a dynamic, multifactorial model. No unmarried chance aspect debts for any or any volatility. A viable causal version would involve biological and psychological diathesis that deal with multiple environmental stressors. There is no doubt that early-onset is carefully linked to grownup recurrence, whether the effects come from research samples, long-term demographic research, high college scholar research, or pressured patient studies. Within five years, approximately 50 percent of suicidal young adults have a recurrence, but most effective a small variety of them did have extreme psychopathology in 365 days. The few findings that tracked suicidal youth into adulthood suggest clear continuity between teenage and grownup melancholy and expanded danger of suicide attempts, as well as mental and surgical hospitalization. Prepubertal melancholy findings indicate continuity in puberty. The worst result is a suicide, the 1/3 main motive of sweet sixteen death. Other results encompass loss of social boom and capabilities, peer withdrawal, low faculty fulfillment, under-most useful task and marriage selections, and drug abuse). This chapter reviews baby and adolescent epidemiology and concepts of temper problems. Also addressed are psychological, social, and organic causes determined to raise the danger of mood disturbances in children and children.

2.1 Depression

For numerous years, children and young adults were taken into consideration unlikely to sense depressed. Thus despair became called "grownup infection." But, as early as the 17th century, case reports identified young adults with signs same to the ones determined in human beings with depressive problems. 1975, State Psychiatric Institution

Health (NIMH) organized a assembly of thinkers to talk about kid's occurrence and diagnosis of depression. This conference, accompanied with the aid of Shulterbrant and Ruskin's e-book, finally defined the proper analysis and despair on this populace.

The ultimate two many years experienced a burgeoning database on the technology of temper disorders. Severe depressive disorder (MDD) is now not visible solely as a center-elderly and elderly ailment. Epidemiological and psychiatric evidence from the United States and abroad has hooked up explicitly that the primary onset age of extensive despair is common in puberty and younger adulthood, and prepubertal onset occurs, albeit less not unusual. Adolescent depression is now evidently a persistent, routine, and dangerous circumstance. Depressed dad and mom' descendants, relative to children with non-depressed dad and mom, have a 2- to four-fold expanded risk of melancholy. Depressions in teenagers share not unusual characteristics with depression at other a long time. Symptom traits are commonplace across intervals; woman fees are higher (2-fold hazard); high comorbidity of anxiety issues, drug dependence, and suicidal behaviors; elevated social, occupational, and academic impairment can accompany depression. Conversely, youth

MDD seems to be overwhelmingly male, temper-reactive, and normally related to expanded ranges of irritability and dysphonia, and has a tendency to be rather comorbid with disruptive behavioral problems. Epidemiological records on childhood and adolescent bipolar sickness are drastically sparser than MDD records, in part due to the sooner inaccurate assumption that bipolar disease takes place in adulthood. Also, it's far too complex to pick out distinctions among normal temper and irritability in teens, specifically in organization research, and the first indications of bipolar sickness are usually unclear. Much proof of sweet sixteen bipolar ailment comes from research studies wherein tries had been made, particularly currently, to classify the early medical bipolar disorder.

Unfortunately, human beings underneath 18 have been exempt from epidemiological trials earlier than these days. Empirically-based facts on occurrence, chance elements, route, and remedy is, therefore, scanty, in particular for bipolar disorder. This situation is slowly improving, but not quickly enough; temper problems often have profound implications for the destiny development of education, employment, marriage, and the following technology. This bankruptcy highlights the medical basis for explaining early life epidemiology, phenomenology, route, and comorbidity of MDD and bipolar sickness. Since a pointy difference can't be made among youth and teenage onset, childhood (prepubertal-onset) situation details might be used where appropriate.

Diagnosis of the equal standards diagnosed within the Psychiatric Disorders Diagnostic and Statistical Manual to diagnose adult MDD is used to diagnose teenage MDD. During the equal 2-week period, five or six of the following symptoms have to seem almost every day to analysis a teenager with a primary depressive episode:

• Sad or irritated temper maximum days

• Lost hobby or enjoyment in almost all sports activities, maximum of the day

• Major weight loss, advantage, or urge for food trade; inability to advantage anticipated weight

• Sleep disorder

• Psychomotor agitation or pause

• Fatigue or electricity loss

• Inappropriate disgrace or hopelessness

• Indecisiveness or decreased focus

• Frequent demise or suicidal ideation, suicide try.

At least certainly one of signs should be gift: careworn or irritable mood, or notably reduced involvement or pride in without a doubt all duties. These symptoms must purpose clinically relevant dysfunction in social, occupational, or different critical functional environments. They can not be attributed to the overt neurological effect of opioid addiction or preferred medical ailment. Often, grief or schizoaffective confusion ought to no longer better account for signs and symptoms. A fundamental depressive contamination cannot be superimposed over undefined dementia, schizophreniform ailment, delusional disease, or psychotic condition. MDD can be categorised as moderate, slight, or intense, with or without psychotic signs and symptoms, incomplete or partial remission. Depression may be recognized as continual until the episode reaches two successive years. Furthermore, whether or not there may be a loss of enjoyment in almost all responsibilities or a lack of reactivity to generally fulfilling sensations, the disease may also have melancholic traits. Moreover, depression includes at the least 3 of the following:

• Sad state, noticeably unique from the lack of a cherished one

• Early unhappiness is worse than day or night

• Several hours earlier than normal

• Evident psychomotor postpone or anxiety

• Major loss or anorexia

• Deficient or useless disgrace

To outline a psychotic episode as catatonic, ought to be present:

• Immobility, catalepsy, or stupor

• Objective motor over pastime, no longer in response to the outside stimulus

• Strong negativism.

• Curiosities which includes posturing, grimacing, stereotyping, and mannerisms echolalia

Determining mood ailment's seasonality is regularly complicated but additionally sizable considering a major depressive episode can first of all seem in youngsters and youth as a seasonal affective disorder. To create a real temper disorder, there need to be a everyday temporal association between mood disease (depression or mania) and a particular time of 12 months. Complete remission or alternate from depression to obsession should arise throughout that unmarried yr. The teen nonetheless has to undergo two mood sickness episodes over the last years, and the seasonal episodes can outnumber no seasonal episodes. The seasonal temper disturbance is frequently unnoticed in teens due to the uncertainty of starting a new academic year in autumn. Postpartum despair in young adults is taken into consideration as depression starts offevolved inside four weeks of childbirth. Another frequently undetected sickness in young adults is dysthymia, defined in young people because the depressed or irritable mood that have to be gift for a yr or longer. The children ought to in no way be freed from symptoms for greater than months.